2016 年度
药品检查报告

国家食品药品监督管理总局
年度检查报告系列

国家食品药品监督管理总局
食品药品审核查验中心
CENTER FOR FOOD AND DRUG INSPECTION OF CFDA

中国医药科技出版社

图书在版编目（CIP）数据

2016 年度药品检查报告 / 国家食品药品监督管理总局食品药品审核查验中心编 . — 北京：中国医药科技出版社，2017.12

（国家食品药品监督管理总局年度检查报告系列）

ISBN 978-7-5067-9772-6

Ⅰ . ① 2…　Ⅱ . ①国…　Ⅲ . ①药品 – 检查 – 调查报告 – 2016　Ⅳ . ① R97

中国版本图书馆 CIP 数据核字 (2017) 第 287837 号

美术编辑　陈君杞

版式设计　锋尚设计

出版　中国医药科技出版社

地址　北京市海淀区文慧园北路甲 22 号

邮编　100082

电话　发行：010–62227427 邮购：010–62236938

网址　www.cmstp.com

规格　787 × 1092mm　$\frac{1}{16}$

印张　$5\frac{3}{4}$

字数　97 千字

版次　2017 年 12 月第 1 版

印次　2017 年 12 月第 1 次印刷

印刷　北京瑞禾彩色印刷有限公司

经销　全国各地新华书店

书号　ISBN 978-7-5067-9772-6

定价　48.00 元

编委会

序

在国家食品药品监督管理总局的坚强领导下，2016年国家食品药品监督管理总局食品药品审核查验中心完成了药品注册生产现场检查、药品GMP认证检查、药品GMP跟踪检查、飞行检查、进口药品境外生产现场检查、流通检查以及观察检查等各类检查。本报告包括中英文版，阐述了2016年药品检查情况及检查发现的主要问题，分析了各类检查发现的薄弱环节和潜在质量风险。

2016年国家药品检查工作有效开展，发现和处置问题能力进一步提高，有力震慑了违法违规行为，在保障公众用药安全中发挥了重要作用。

国家食品药品监督管理总局食品药品审核查验中心

二〇一七年五月

前 言

食品药品审核查验中心全年组织开展药品注册生产现场检查、药品GMP认证检查、GMP跟踪检查、飞行检查、进口药品境外生产现场检查、流通检查以及观察检查共计431项。

2016 年完成各类药品检查任务一览表

检查工作	检查企业数/品种数	派出组数	派出人次
药品注册生产现场检查	34	43	178
药品GMP认证检查	16	16	47
药品GMP跟踪检查	204	197	704
药品飞行检查	39	39	155
进口药品境外生产现场检查	7	7	31
药品流通检查	50	50	77
国际观察检查	81	81	85
合计	431	433	1277

目 录

第一章
药品注册生产现场检查

一、检查基本情况

2016年共收到29个检查任务（包括多阶段检查），21个来自总局药品审评中心（以下简称"药审中心"），8个有因检查任务。共派出43个检查组178人次对34个品规进行了现场检查；完成现场检查报告42个，其中通过34个，占81%；不通过及企业主动撤回注册申请的8个，占19%。

表 1-1 现场检查派组情况

检查总数（品规）	检查组数	检查员人次
34	43	178

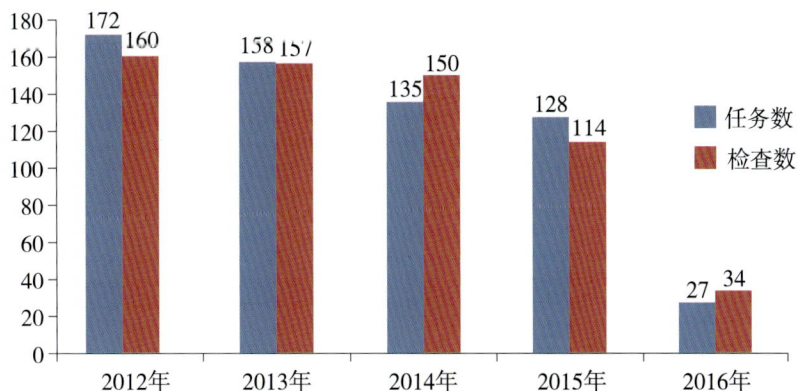

图1-1 近五年药品注册生产现场检查任务数量图

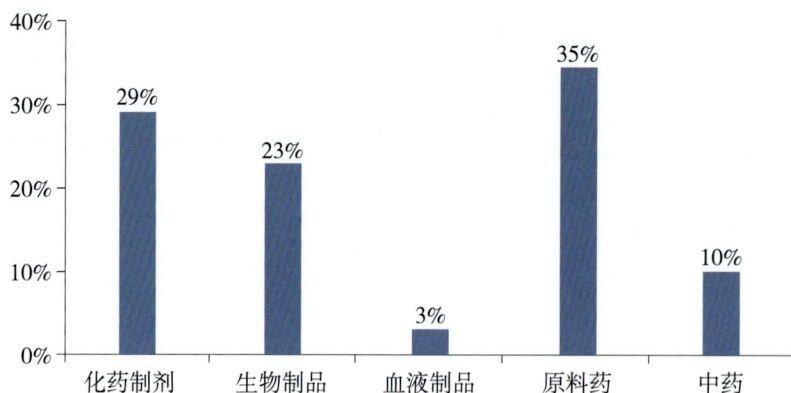

图1-2　现场检查剂型分布图

二、发现主要问题

在2016年的现场检查中，个别企业的数据无法溯源、申报资料不真实等数据可靠性问题仍然突出，同时发现工艺验证不充分、生产工艺不稳定、生产工艺或参数与核定的不一致等问题。

具体情况如下：

（一）数据可靠性问题

（1）检验数据不能溯源。没有按规定留样并进行稳定性考察。现场检查未见检查品种试制样品的留样和稳定性试验留样，也不能提供相应记录。

（2）批生产记录不真实、不完整，与申报资料不符。

（二）工艺验证不充分，生产工艺不稳定

品种的工艺验证不充分，企业在动态生产时，出现严重偏差、批量生产收率与验证批次的偏离较大、生产设备控制系统不稳定、生产线的部分设备不能完全满足现有生产要求。

（三）生产工艺或关键工艺参数、内包材与核定内容不一致，未进行研究评估

（1）生产工艺与核定的/申报的生产工艺不一致。

（2）关键工艺参数与核定的/申报的生产工艺不一致。

（3）内包材生产商与注册申报不一致，企业未进行对比研究。

（四）未进行必要的偏差调查

动态生产中出现重大异常情况时，个别企业调查不充分，找不到根本原因。某化学原料药工艺验证三批和动态生产批结果显示，4批成品收率差距较大，企业没有分析查找原因。

第二章
药品 GMP 认证检查

一、检查基本情况

依据国家食品药品监督管理总局关于"未通过药品生产质量管理规范（2010年修订）认证企业停止生产和下放无菌药品认证有关事宜的公告（2015年第285号）"的精神，自2016年1月1日起，国家食品药品监督管理总局不再受理药品GMP认证申请。对于已经受理的认证申请，继续组织完成现场检查和审核发证。

鉴于上述情况，2016年全年共安排检查16家，接收现场检查报告16份，完成审核件14份，其中12家药品生产企业通过药品GMP认证检查，2家药品生产企业未通过药品GMP认证检查，发出告诫信的企业5家；另有2家企业其GMP认证检查虽然结束，但因尚未拿到相关注册批准证明性文件，认证程序暂停。

申请认证的剂型包括大容量注射剂3家次、小容量注射剂3家次、冻干粉针剂3家次、粉针剂1家次、放射性药品1家次、疫苗类产品2家次、其他类生物制品3家次。

表 2-1 现场检查派组情况

检查总数	检查组数	检查员人次
16	16	47

表 2-2 2016 年认证检查剂型分布情况（单位：家次）

大容量注射剂	小容量注射剂	冻干粉针剂	粉针剂	放射性药品	疫苗	生物制品（其他）
3	3	3	1	1	2	3

二、发现主要问题

发现220条缺陷，包括主要缺陷23项，一般缺陷197项。其中质量控制与质量保证方面41项，文件管理方面缺陷32项，机构与人员方面缺陷24项，设备方面缺陷23项，确认与验证方面缺陷21项。与2015年检查发现缺陷的分布基本一致。

本年度认证检查的两家体外诊断试剂生产企业，结果均为不通过，主要问题如下：

1. 质量管理体系方面

质量管理体系不能有效运行，无法保证产品的生产和质量要求；人员流动性大，专业人员欠缺，培训不到位，无法满足日常生产质量管理要求；文件可操作性不强，数据记录不完整；相关变更没有按照变更程序进行变更控制。

2. 确认与验证工作方面

未对所有申请GMP认证的产品进行工艺验证，对公用设备设施的清洁验证工作不到位；部分验证记录不完整；部分再验证工作未按要求开展等。

第三章
药品 GMP 跟踪检查

一、检查基本情况

　　2016年核查中心公告跟踪检查计划215家，共计228家次。其中停产、长期不生产等企业58家次，其余170家次全部进行了检查。另外，对省级认证的无菌药品生产企业21家进行跟踪检查，双随机检查13家。全年共完成跟踪检查204家次。

表 3-1　检查派组情况

检查总数（家次）	检查组数	检查员人次
204	197	704

表 3-2　检查分布情况

类别	计划检查数量	实际检查数量
2015年度抽验不合格的企业	11	10
2015年发放告诫信的企业	37	32
疫苗生产企业	38	36
血液制品生产企业	28	25
高风险品种生产企业	114	67
省级认证的无菌药品生产企业	21	21

类别	计划检查数量	实际检查数量
双随机检查	13	13
共计	262	204

跟踪检查不通过的企业有12家，占6.1%，发告诫信的企业有59家，占29.6%。

在检查不通过的12家企业中，2015年度抽验不合格的企业有5家，双随机检查的企业4家，胞磷胆碱钠注射剂生产企业2家，骨肽注射剂生产企业1家。

（一）2015 年度质量公告品种抽查情况

共对10家企业进行了跟踪检查，其中5家检查不通过，占50%，另对4家企业发放告诫信。

（二）双随机检查

为落实国务院创新事中、事后监管的要求，按照总局统一部署，药品双随机检查系统于2016年12月首次运行，采取分层双随机的方法对选出的13家企业开展了跟踪检查，包括化学制剂3个、原料药2个、中药8个，分布在9个省。共有4家企业检查不通过，通过率仅69%，另对3家企业发告诫信。

（三）疫苗生产企业

对获得药品GMP证书的38家疫苗生产企业列入2016年跟踪检查计划，除1家因药品生产许可证和药品GMP证书于2014年收回、1家因2015年申请变更生产地址药品GMP证书未拿到没有执行检查外，共对36家疫苗生产企业进行了跟踪检查。检查结果全部通过，共对7家企业发告诫信。其中一家企业因变更分析检测器，检查组现场初步认为属严重缺陷，后期专家研讨认为变更前后的检测器方法原理一致，质量风险较低，要求企业开展进一步的方法学对比验证，降为主要缺陷。总体来说，疫苗生产质量风险可控，生产企业的生产和质量管理较规范。

（四）血液制品生产企业

26家血液制品生产企业列入2016年跟踪检查计划，共对25家血液制品企业开展跟踪检查，另有1家企业因停产整改未进行检查。检查结果全部通过，共对4家企业发告诫信。总体来说，我国血液制品生产质量风险可控，生产企业的生产和质量管理较规范，对个别企业仍需加强监管力度。

（五）2015 年发告诫信的企业

共对2015年发告诫信的32家企业进行了跟踪检查，尽管企业基本符合要求，但仍对14家企业再次发告诫信。

（六）认证下放后，对省级认证的无菌药品生产企业抽查情况

共抽查省级认证的无菌药品生产企业21家，全部通过，对其中6家企业发告诫信。通过抽查，省局认证检查的尺度总体把握严格，各地平稳承接了下放的认证检查职能。

（七）高风险品种的专项检查

本年度重点对骨肽、果糖二磷酸钠、胞磷胆碱钠等三个产品的注射剂进行了跟踪检查，计划进行114家次的高风险品种专项检查，其中有47家因企业未通过药品GMP（2010年修订）认证、品种长期停产、批准文号转移等原因未进行检查，实际检查67家次。1家骨肽注射剂生产企业和2家胞磷胆碱钠注射剂生产企业不通过，对21家企业发告诫信。

二、发现主要问题

（一）总体情况

204家次检查共发现2260条缺陷项，其中严重缺陷22项，主要缺陷212项，一般缺陷2026项，与2015年GMP认证、跟踪检查相比严重缺陷数目有所增加。

在高风险品种专项检查的企业中品种长期停产或未通过药品GMP（2010年

修订）认证的现象比较突出，检查发现的一些共性问题如下：

（1）个别存在生产工艺与注册工艺不一致问题。

（2）数据可靠性问题仍然存在，包括伪造生产记录，检验记录中套用图谱、擅自修改数据问题，生产、设备、物料记录中相关内容不符等问题。

（3）工艺验证不充分，特别是变更生产批量后未进行工艺验证的问题较多。

（4）数据管理的规范性问题突出，主要体现在系统权限设置、审计追踪功能、文件和数据的修改及删除权限等未进行控制，以及对删除数据和选择使用的数据没有合理控制和解释。

（5）计算机化系统、确认和验证两个附录的实施情况与法规要求存在一定差距，发现问题较多。

（6）对偏差和变更的管理较薄弱，主要体现在对发生的偏差不能有效识别并记录，对变更缺少必要的评估和验证。

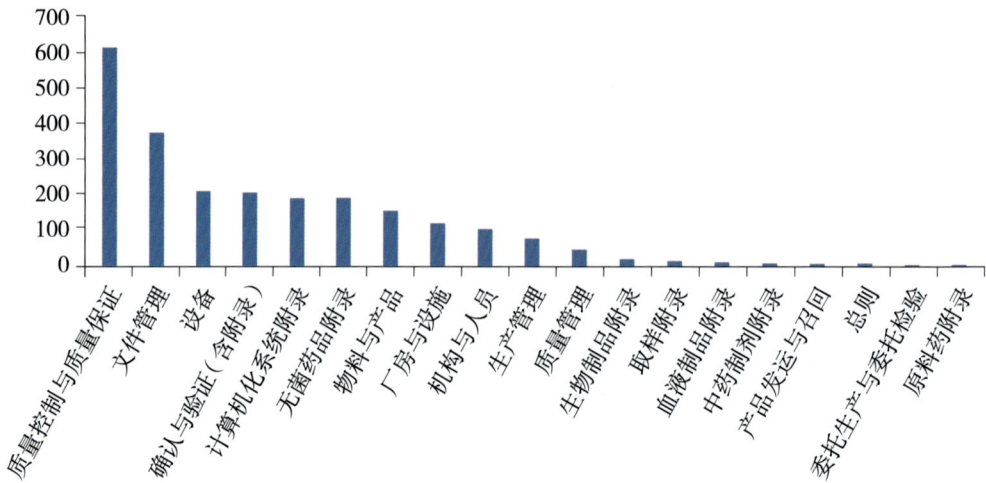

图3-1　跟踪检查缺陷项目分布情况

（二）2015 年度抽验不合格的企业

检查10家企业共发现严重缺陷11项，主要缺陷27项，一般缺陷84项。

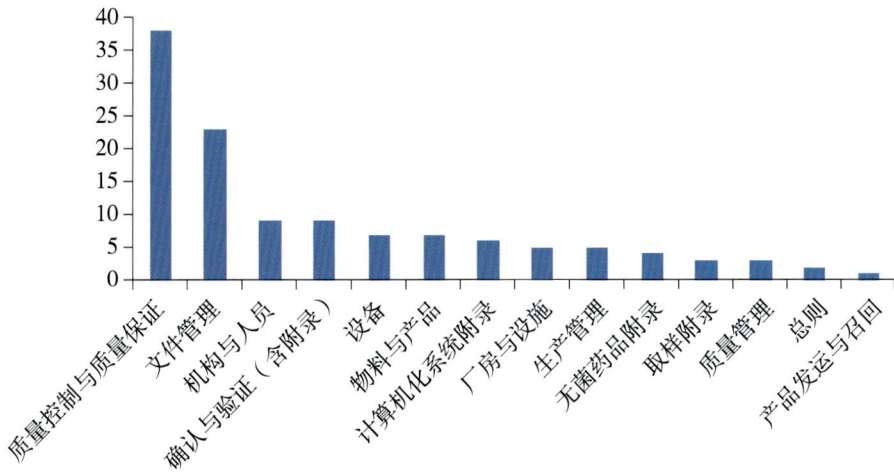

图3-2　抽验不合格企业缺陷项目分布情况

发现的主要问题包括：生产工艺与注册工艺不一致，数据可靠性问题，工艺验证问题。

（三）双随机检查

发现严重缺陷5项，主要缺陷24项，一般缺陷123项。

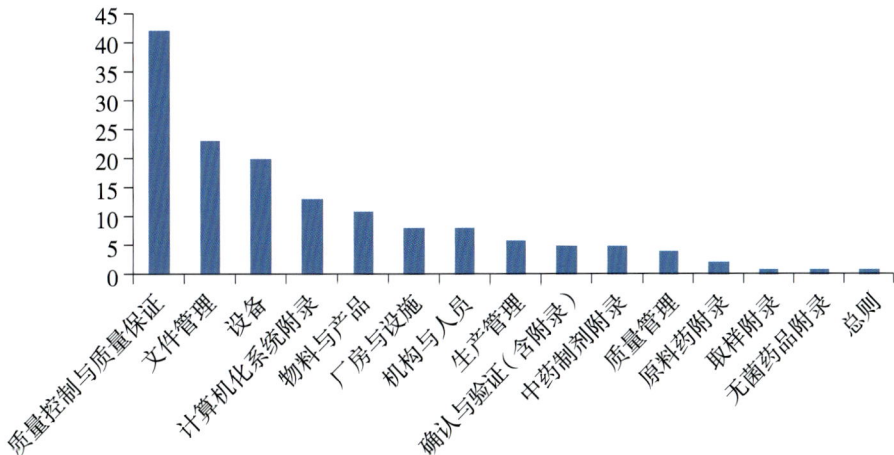

图3-3　双随机检查缺陷项目分布情况

发现的主要问题包括：伪造记录，产品存在质量安全隐患，数据可靠性问题，工艺验证存在问题，物料管理不规范，存在污染、混淆和差错风险，清洁不彻底，不能有效防止污染和交叉污染。

（四）疫苗生产企业

发现主要缺陷38项，一般缺陷383项。

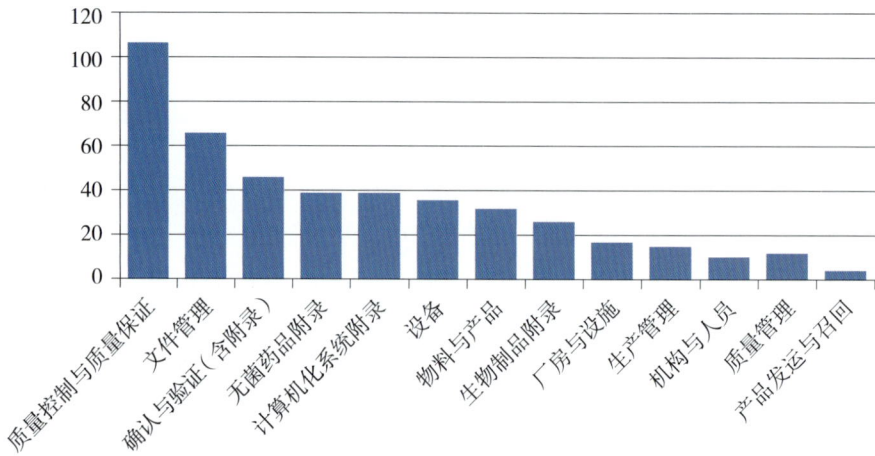

图3-4　疫苗生产企业检查缺陷项目分布情况

发现的主要问题包括：

1．设备方面

注射用水制备系统进入注射水储罐的不锈钢管路阀门到制水机之间过长。

2．物料与产品方面

成品不合格品销毁记录有待细化；个别货位卡缺失；未建立生产用的菌毒种主种子全基因序列的背景资料。

3．文件管理方面

个别文件规定不够具体、操作性不强，文件规定的内容与实际稍有出入；个别记录内容不全面；批生产记录设计内容不合理，实际操作时填写容易造成不及时。

4．质量控制与质量保证方面

（1）质量实验室管理：未向接受委托检验的机构索取必要的检验数据和图谱。

（2）偏差处理：企业偏差处理相关文件的培训、执行不到位；个别偏差未能及时启动调查；少数偏差原因分析和纠正预防措施不到位，对偏差可能引起的对产品质量的潜在影响没有充分评估。

（3）变更控制：变更未按变更流程处理并申报注册补充申请。对某些变更没有进行评估或评估不充分。

（4）供应商管理：对关键物料供应商的审计内容有待细化，供应商审计内容针对性有待提高。

（5）产品质量回顾：应按品种分别进行年度质量回顾，且回顾中对CAPA有效性分析不足；年度产品质量回顾分析报告分析内容可进一步细化。

5．计算机化系统

企业制定了计算机化系统管理的文件制度，但并未完全按照制度分类进行管理，对现有条件不符合文件的情形，未采取有效措施降低风险；质量检验室HPLC检测设备登录界面权限设置要求需细化。

（五）血液制品生产企业

共检查25家企业，发现严重缺陷0项，主要缺陷13项，一般缺陷241项。

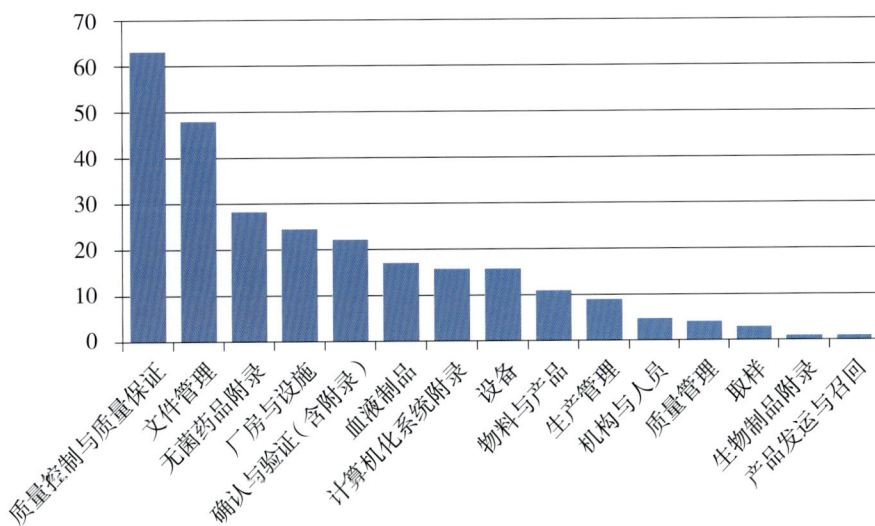

图3-5　血液制品生产企业检查缺陷项目分布情况

发现的主要问题：

1．机构与人员方面

对部分岗位操作人员培训欠缺。

2．厂房与设施方面

存在不能有效控制污染和交叉污染的可能。

3．设备方面

部分设备校准未覆盖实际使用范围；部分检验用仪器设备未定期校准或校准不充分，记录不完善；部分设备标识不全。

4．物料与产品方面

价拨冷沉淀标签中信息不充分，标签未固定。

5．确认与验证方面

培养基模拟灌装实验未明确干预要求、剔除标准等具体要求。

6．文件管理方面

工艺规程、操作程序等文件内容不具体，规定不规范。记录存在不及时填写、填写不全面等不规范行为。

7．生产管理方面

灭活前加入的辛酸钠溶液，缺少微生物的控制措施；未对沉降碟在A级层流下的放置时间进行确认。

8．质量控制与质量保证方面

（1）质控实验室管理：检品收发台账记录内容不完整，未记录中间品、半成品检验样品的接收信息；未对外购的用于环境监测的平皿培养基进行检测；无菌试验未按药典设置阴性对照；

（2）产品稳定性考察：中间产品制定了效期，但缺少持续稳定性考察或验证数据支持；

（3）变更控制：变更控制管理不到位。对部分变更没有进行评估或评估不充分；

（4）偏差处理：个别偏差未能及时启动调查；部分偏差调查及纠正和预防措施不充分；

（5）供应商管理：价拨冷沉淀供应商未纳入企业合格供应商目录；

（6）产品质量回顾：某些信息未纳入年度产品质量回顾中；

（7）产品发运与召回：对批签发样品的发运方式未进行规定；

（8）计算机化系统：计算机化系统的管理文件不完善。QC实验室部分仪器设备无审计追踪功能；某些电子数据导入电脑打印后均没有保存和备份；系统未设置不同层级访问权限，存在数据和系统被修改风险。

（六）2015 年发告诚信的企业

检查32家企业共发现严重缺陷2项，主要缺陷32项，一般缺陷328项。

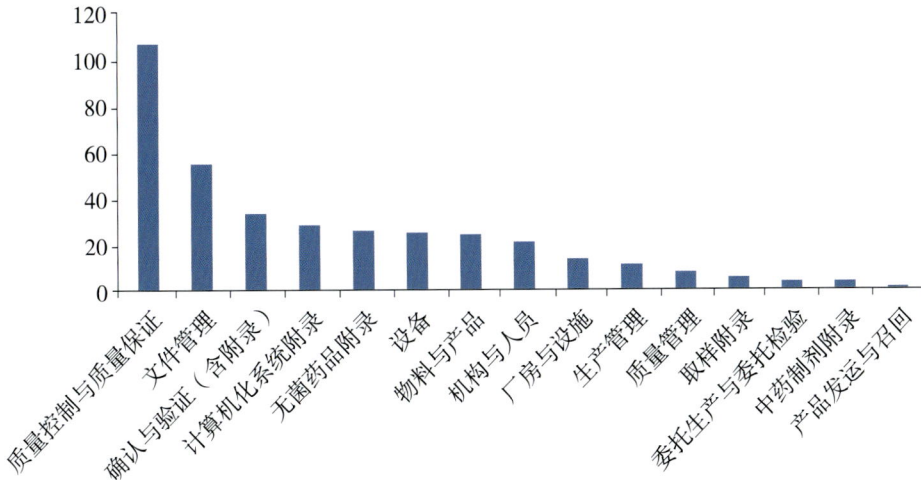

图3-6　2015年发告诚信的企业检查缺陷项目的分布情况

发现的主要问题包括：数据可靠性问题，未对偏差进行记录和调查，无菌保障存在不足，相关确认与验证工作不够充分。

（七）省级认证的无菌药品生产企业

检查21家企业共发现严重缺陷0项，主要缺陷15项，一般缺陷209项。

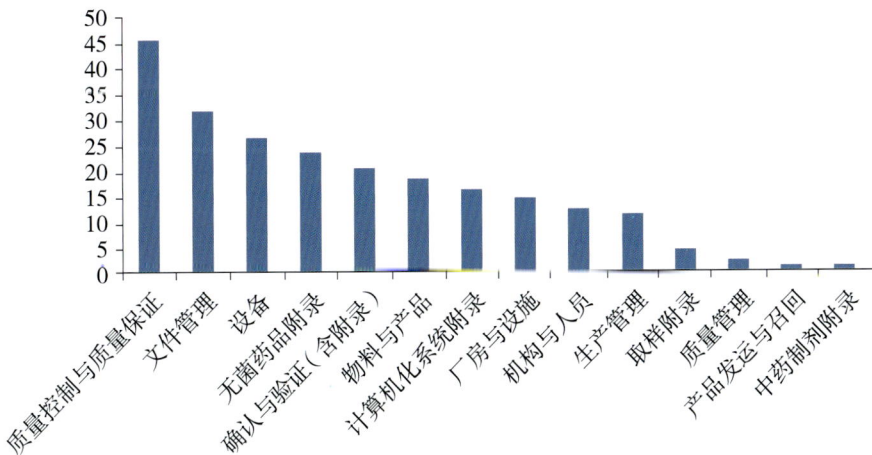

图3-7　省级认证的无菌药品生产企业跟踪检查缺陷项目的分布情况

发现的主要问题表现在：小容量注射剂共线生产风险评估不充分；仅对单品种进行清洁验证，未对企业所有品种进行清洁风险评估；部分检验记录内容不完整；尚未开展计算机化系统的验证和审计工作；物料管理不当，存在混淆、差错风险等。

（八）高风险品种的专项检查

检查61家企业共发现严重缺陷3项，主要缺陷64项，一般缺陷658项。

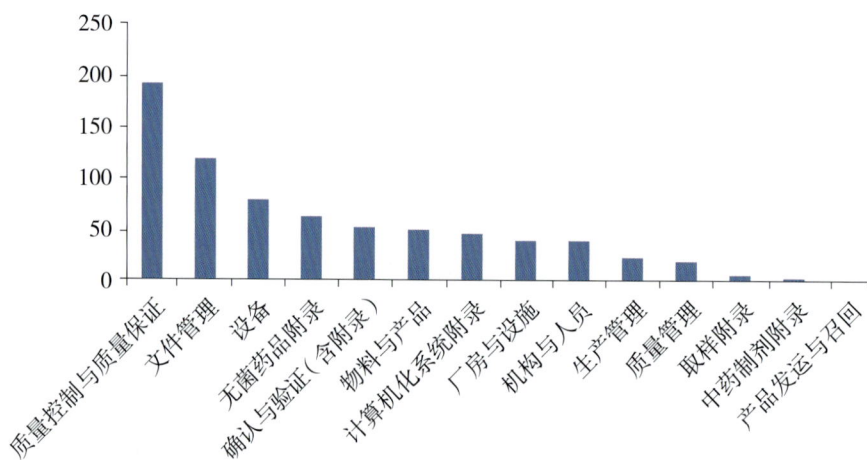

图3-8　高风险品种专项检查缺陷项目分布情况

发现的主要问题如下：

1. 骨肽注射液

（1）从肉制品公司购入的前腿骨，未按规定采购、验收。物料到货后，未按SOP索取、核对供应商出具的检验报告；验收时，未索取猪四肢骨冷链运输温度监测记录。

（2）复方骨肽原溶液的病毒灭活未经验证；对猪四肢骨提取后存放时间、复方骨肽注射液从灌封到灭菌开始的时间没有验证数据支持。

（3）持续稳定性考察方案未对活性指标及相关的安全性指标加以规定及检验，如过敏实验、热原、异常毒性等。

2. 果糖二磷酸钠注射液

果糖二磷酸钠企业内控标准中微生物限度标准未按《中国药典》2015年版

相应规定进行修订；用于果糖二磷酸钠原料药含量测定用的复合酶试剂超过保质期后，仍用于原料药的含量测定。

3. 胞磷胆碱钠注射液

某企业胞磷胆碱钠原料药内控标准制定不合理，未参照原料药生产企业质量标准增加甲苯残留的项目。某企业胞磷胆碱钠注射液未分别对不同厂家的原料进行分开工艺验证；未提供胞磷胆碱钠注射液除菌过滤器相容性试验的相容性试验资料。

第四章
药品飞行检查

一、基本情况

2016年共接收总局飞检任务45次，完成并上报结果的药品GMP飞行检查39家次，其他于2017年开展。已上报结果的39家次中，涉及北京、江苏、广东等20个省（市），共包括9家生化药品生产企业、20家中药生产企业、9家普通化学药品生产企业及1家血液制品生产企业。

2016年的飞行检查任务中来自总局药化监管司的任务33件，来自总局药化注册司等司局的任务共计6件。总局药化监管司的任务占比约85%，是飞行检查任务的主要来源。39次飞行检查中中药占全部飞行检查工作的51%，普通化学药品和生化药品各占23%。2016年飞行检查共有21家药品生产检查不通过，占比约54%。其中有14家企业被建议收回药品GMP证书，10家企业被建议立案调查，7家企业的问题产品被责令召回。在药品GMP飞行检查中，中药和生化药品发现的问题较多。总局已经依法依规对飞行检查中发现的问题进行了处理。

表 4-1　飞行检查处理情况

产品类别	检查家次	不通过	收回GMP证书	产品召回
中药	20	14	9	2
生化药品	9	5	4	4

续表

产品类别	检查家次	不通过	收回GMP证书	产品召回
血液制品	1	1	1	1
普通化药	9	1	0	0

二、发现主要问题

（一）中药类企业发现的主要问题

2016年针对中药类生产企业，共派出18个检查组66人次对20家企业进行了飞行检查，其中涉及信访举报的7家企业，人工牛黄生产企业3家，含牛黄类产品7家企业，探索性研究检验发现问题3家企业，中药饮片1家企业。

20家中药类生产企业的飞行检查，其中12家企业不符合药品GMP要求，对3家企业的有关问题移交省局处理，对1家企业发出了告诫信，1家企业无相关生产，符合要求的有3家企业。

1. 中成药生产企业

（1）擅自改变工艺问题较为突出：中成药口服制剂为降低生产成本，擅自改变前处理、提取工艺的现象还是一个比较突出的问题。本年度因探索性检验发现问题开展飞行检查的，均是企业将处方中部分应提取的中药材不按工艺规程进行提取，而是粉碎后直接投料。

（2）中药材、中药饮片物料管理混乱：个别中成药生产企业，为应对各级药品监督管理部门的监督检查，编造仓库物料台账和出入库记录，根据中成药的生产量倒推出中药材的使用量，并按需用量编造物料台账。

（3）对购入的中药材、中药饮片不能严格全检，且数据可靠性存在问题：传统中成药生产企业产品品种多，涉及的中药材、中药饮片品种也多，由于配置的精密分析仪器和QC人员与生产规模不相适应，不能保证购入的中药材和中药饮片批批全检，造成对部分批次中药材、中药饮片不进行全检，或者采用一图多用的行为应对检查。

2. 人工牛黄

部分企业不能按照药品GMP要求组织生产，尤其是对人工牛黄上游产业链供应商审计和管理要求严重不足，供应商的加工场所卫生环境恶劣，原材料来源无法溯源，加工过程不可控。主要问题包括：①供应商管理环节薄弱；②微生物限度检查结果真实性存疑；③未纳入质量保证体系。

3. 中药饮片

购进中药材或炮制后产品的含量检测问题突出，染色、增重问题时有发生，批生产记录真实性存疑。主要问题包括：①批生产记录不真实；②涉嫌外购饮片进行分装、销售；③数据可靠性问题。

（二）生化药品

1. "单唾液酸四己糖神经节苷酯钠"的检查

2016年共检查4家"单唾液酸四己糖神经节苷酯钠"生产企业，发现其在原料质量和供应商管理方面存在一定的风险。主要问题包括：

（1）供应商管理有待提高，企业对供应商的管理不能保证有效的追溯性。

（2）对原料冷链运输监控的电子数据管理不够。

2. "注射用促肝细胞生长素"的检查

2016年共检查4家"注射用促肝细胞生长素"生产企业，其中2家企业被收回药品GMP证书，对另外2家企业发出了告诫信。主要问题包括：①编造记录文件；②数据可靠性问题；③与注册生产工艺不一致；④无法有效保证肝脏原料的质量。

第五章
进口药品境外检查

一、检查基本情况

（一）年度检查任务概况

按照总局《关于执行2016年度进口药品境外生产现场检查计划的函》等文件要求。2016年度境外任务共计49个。

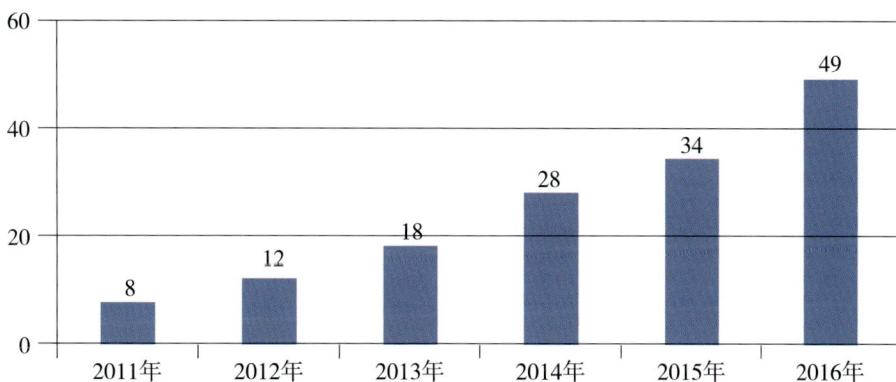

图5-1　2011～2016年境外检查任务量

（1）2016年检查任务涉及19个国家。其中欧洲、北美等地区品种数量居多，药品质量地域性风险高的印度、越南等国家的检查品种也占一定比例，同时增加对南美地区和澳洲地区检查力度。

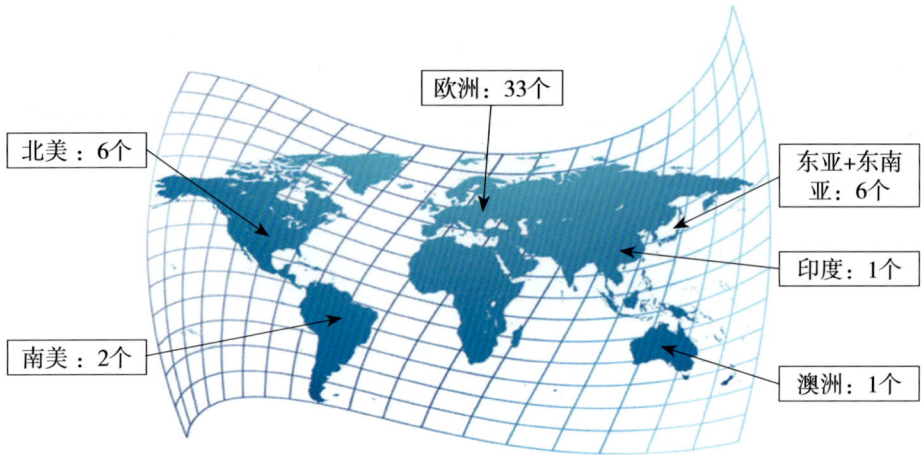

图5-2　2016年计划检查任务国家分布情况

（2）遵循检查服务于审评审批的原则，兼顾已上市产品安全要求，在审品种检查比例增大，申报临床、申报生产、再注册和补充申请阶段产品均纳入检查范围，已上市产品检查的原因主要为口岸质量检验问题，增加不良反应监测风险较高品种。

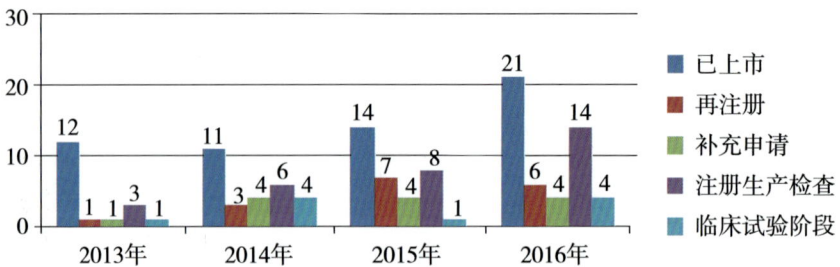

图5-3　近年检查任务注册状态

（3）检查任务显现品种全面、剂型广泛等特点，并加大对化学药品制剂的延伸检查力度。涉及化学药品40个，含注射剂、固体制剂、植入剂、鼻喷剂等，其中生化药3个，延伸检查原料药6个；疫苗、血液制品、治疗用生物制品11个；植物药4个。

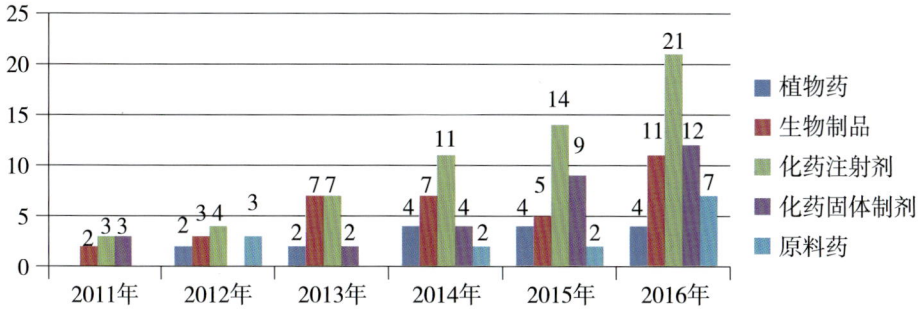

图5-4　检查任务分类情况

（二）2016年检查执行情况

由于年中总局工作安排，重新调整了2016年境外检查计划时间，生产企业排产变化导致2016年共完成15个品种检查任务，其中赴现场检查7个品种，3个品种不通过，占检查数量的42%；8个品种在检查组织期间，企业主动撤销品种进口注册证，或被退审等，占年度总计划的17%。另21个品种由于企业排产原因，于2017年第一季度完成检查，剩余12个品种，因企业无法在2017年第一季度接受检查，已纳入2017年境外检查计划。

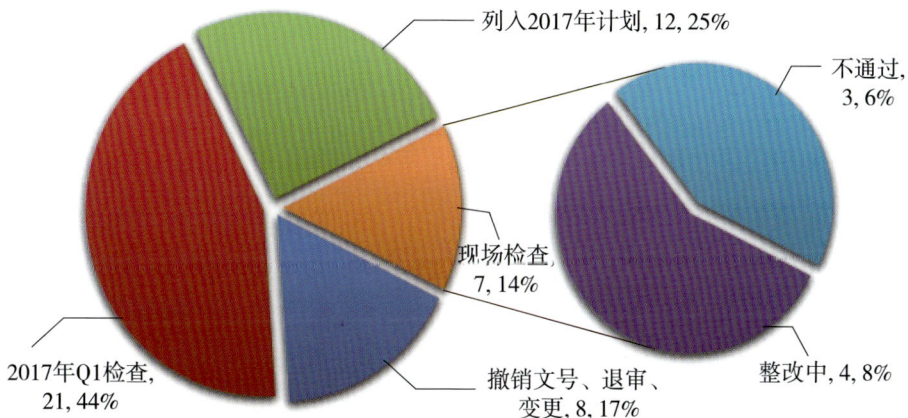

图5-5　2016年检查开展情况

二、境外检查发现主要问题

已检查的7个品种中，3个品种不通过，不通过率较往年有所提高。检查共发现缺陷117项，其中严重缺陷3项，主要缺陷18项。问题主要集中在质量控制与质量保证、物料系统、变更管理等方面；严重缺陷主要为生产工艺一致性以及数据可靠性问题。对境外发现的问题都依法依规进行处理。

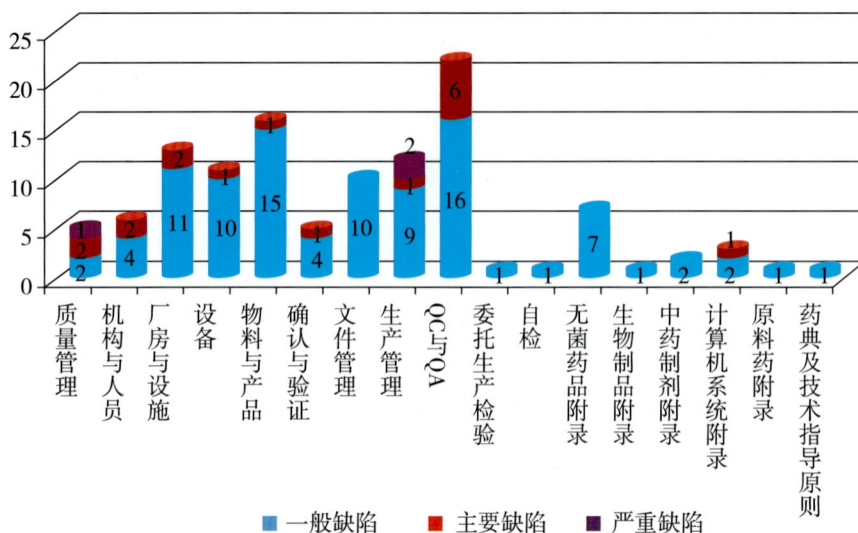

图5-6　2016年境外检查发现缺陷汇总分析

主要及严重问题如下：

（1）实际生产工艺、生产场地等与注册申报不一致，重大变更等情况未向我国进行申报却已执行。

（2）数据可靠性存在重大问题，严重影响产品质量。

（3）非现场检查处理品种数量增多。

第六章
药品流通检查

一、检查基本情况

2016年度，国家食品药品监督管理总局对药品流通领域违法经营行为开展了集中整治，通过企业自查整改，省局监督检查，总局实施飞检等方式进一步整顿和规范药品流通秩序，严厉打击违法经营行为。全年共组织3批，对50家药品批发企业进行了检查。飞行检查结果由总局对外进行公告。

表 6-1　2016 年度药品流通检查任务情况

飞行批次	检查企业数（家）	派出人数（人次）
第一批	28	37
第二批	11	20
第三批	11	20
总计	50	77

检查组依据《总局关于整治药品流通领域违法经营行为的公告》（2016年第94号）以及《药品经营质量管理规范》对相关企业进行了飞行检查。结果发现，药品流通企业存在的违法违规行为较为普遍，情况如下。

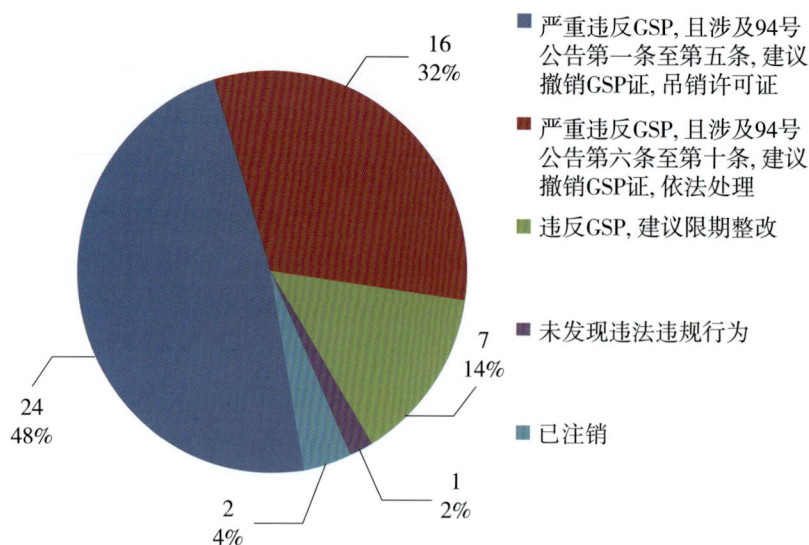

严重违反GSP，且涉及94号公告第一条至第五条，建议撤销GSP证，吊销许可证

严重违反GSP，且涉及94号公告第六条至第十条，建议撤销GSP证，依法处理

违反GSP，建议限期整改

未发现违法违规行为

已注销

图6-1   50家药品批发企业飞行检查结果

二、发现主要问题

（一）企业违反总局 94 号公告情况

表 6-2   药品流通领域飞行检查企业违反 94 号公告情况

94号公告相关条款	涉嫌违反企业数	比例
（一）为他人违法经营药品提供场所、资质证明文件、票据等条件	10家	20%
（二）从个人或者无《药品生产许可证》《药品经营许可证》的单位购进药品	1家	2%
（三）向无合法资质的单位或者个人销售药品，向药品零售企业销售疫苗，知道或者应当知道他人从事无证经营仍为其提供药品	1家	2%
（四）伪造药品采购来源，虚构药品销售流向，篡改计算机系统、温湿度监测系统数据，隐瞒真实药品购销存记录、票据、凭证、数据等，药品购销存记录不完整、不真实，经营行为无法追溯	16家	32%
（五）购销药品时，证（许可证书）、票（发票、随货同行票据）、账（实物账、财务账）、货（药品实物）、款（货款）不能相互对应一致；药品未入库，设立账外账，药品未纳入企业质量体系管理，使用银行个人账户进行业务往来等情形	19家	38%

94号公告相关条款	涉嫌违反企业数	比例
（六）将麻醉药品、精神药品和含特殊药品复方制剂流入非法渠道，或者进行现金交易	3家	6%
（七）在核准地址以外的场所储存药品	6家	12%
（八）未按规定对药品储存、运输、进行温湿度监测	21家	42%
（九）擅自改变注册地址、经营方式、经营范围销售药品	5家	10%
（十）向药品零售企业、诊所销售药品未做到开具销售发票且随货同行	6家	12%

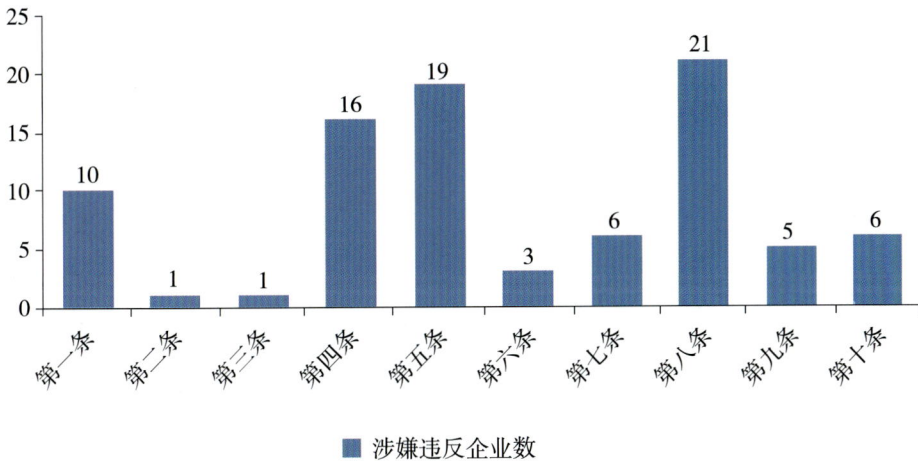

图6-2　企业违反94号公告条款分布情况

存在主要问题：

（1）未按规定对药品储存、运输、进行温湿度监测。

（2）购销药品时，证（许可证书）、票（发票、随货同行票据）、账（实物账、财务账）、货（药品实物）、款（货款）不能相互对应一致；药品未入库，设立账外账，药品未纳入企业质量体系管理，使用银行个人账户进行业务往来等情形。

（3）伪造药品采购来源，虚构药品销售流向，篡改计算机系统、温湿度监

测系统数据，隐瞒真实药品购销存记录、票据、凭证、数据等，药品购销存记录
不完整、不真实，经营行为无法追溯。

（二）企业违反总局药品经营质量管理规范（GSP）情况

表 6-3　药品流通领域飞行检查企业 GSP 缺陷项目分布情况

	**严重缺陷项	*主要缺陷项	总计	比例
总则	35	0	35	16.99%
质量管理体系	0	8	8	3.88%
机构和质量管理职责	0	17	17	8.25%
人员与培训	0	9	9	4.37%
质量管理体系文件	5	6	11	5.34%
设施与设备	0	19	19	9.22%
校准与验证	0	19	19	9.22%
计算机系统	6	9	15	7.28%
采购	2	9	11	5.34%
收货与验收	0	12	12	5.83%
储存与养护	0	23	23	11.17%
销售	18	5	23	11.17%
出库	0	0	0	0.00%
运输与配送	0	3	3	1.46%
售后管理	0	1	1	0.49%
总计	66	140	206	

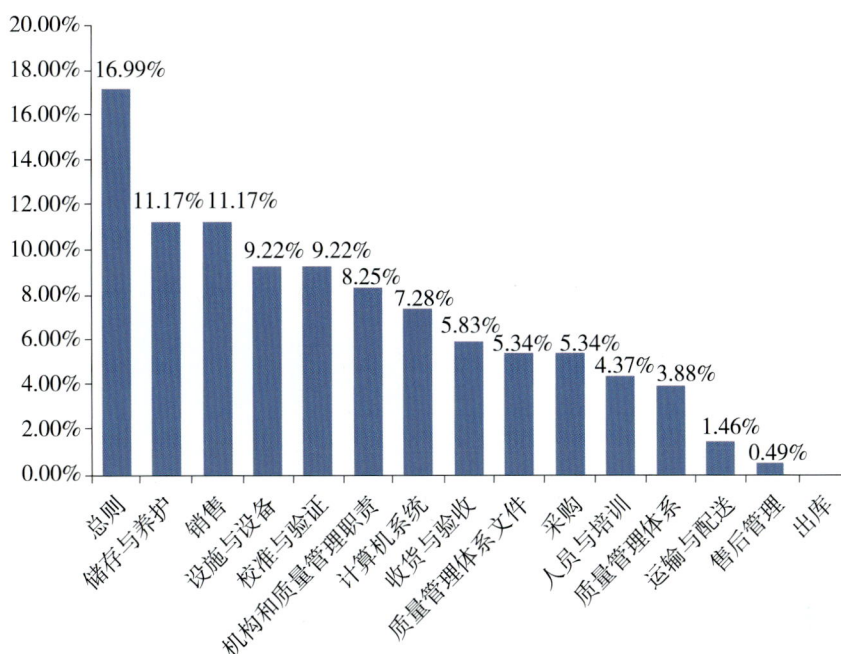

图6-3　企业违反GSP缺陷分布情况

　　药品流通企业GSP缺陷主要集中于总则、储存与养护、销售等方面。主要存在问题：

　　（1）未依法经营，存在虚假、欺骗行为：企业擅自变更经营注册地址；在经营许可范围外设仓库储存药品；为他人违法经营药品提供条件；虚构药品采购来源及销售流向；藏匿票据、提供虚假资料；自查报告不真实；纳税申报表造假；篡改温湿度监测数据等。

　　（2）未按规定储存药品，未对库房温湿度进行有效监测、调控。

　　（3）购销药品吋，票、账、货、款不一致，特药销售未执行国家规定。

第七章
国外机构 GMP 观察检查

一、检查基本情况

2016年核查中心共组织完成药品生产企业的观察检查81家次，涉及企业76家，涵盖浙江、山东等20个省（市），其中浙江、山东、江苏、广东、湖北、海南、河北占80%，与上年度相比基本一致，但各省之间比例略有变化。

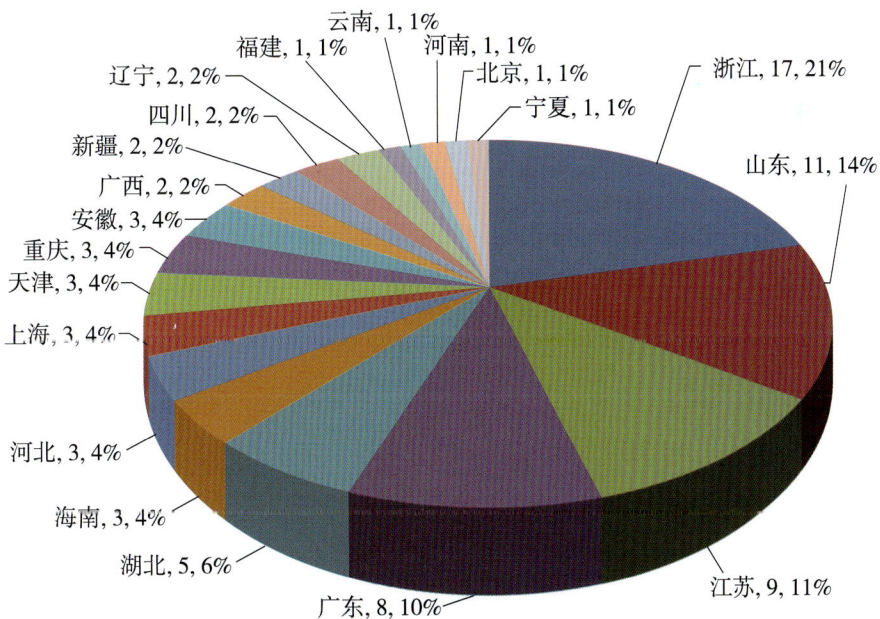

图7-1　2016年国外药品检查观察各省市分布情况

2016年检查观察涉及的检查机构包括世界卫生组织（WHO）、欧洲药品质量理事会（EDQM）、美国食品药品管理局（US FDA）、德国汉堡健康及消费者保护部（BGV）、巴西卫生监督局（ANVISA）、法国国家医药健康安全管理局（ANSM）等12个国际组织或国外药品监管部门。其中发现9家制药企业出现严重缺陷，未通过国外监管/检查机构的现场检查（占比约11%）。

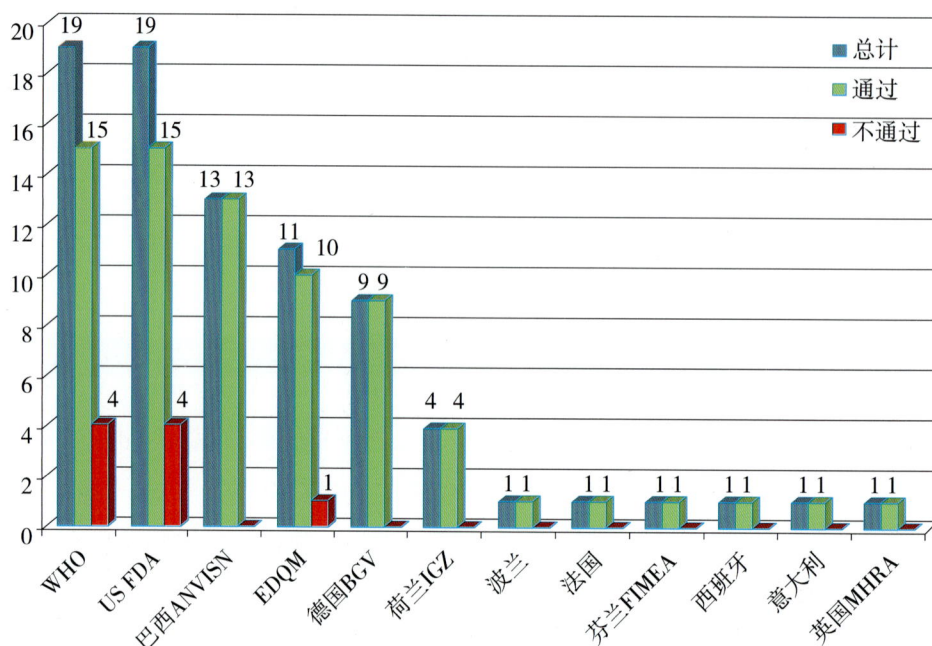

图7-2　2016年国外药品检查观察中不通过情况

　　与2015年相比，不通过比率有所上升。在9家未通过检查的企业中，多数严重缺陷项均涉及数据可靠性问题（包括重复测试至合格、修改系统时间后检测、删除数据、删除审计追踪记录、选择性使用数据、修改电子数据名称、试进样、记录不及时、记录不真实、数据和记录缺失、文件记录控制不足等），部分企业涉及物料标准制定不合理、避免交叉污染的措施不足等方面。总体上，数据可靠性问题较为突出，这也是2016年国内企业接受国外检查不通过率上升的主要原因，也体现出目前药品检查的变化趋势。

　　本年度观察检查共涉及172个药品，包括119个原料药、23个口服固体制剂、19个注射剂、5个生物制品。在81家次检查中涉及原料药的检查共62次，约占全部检查次数的69%，涉及口服固体制剂的检查12次，约占全部检查次数13%。其中原料药占比最大，其次是口服固体制剂，其他剂型出口相对较少。

与2015年相比，其他剂型（包括无菌制剂、生物制品等）接受检查的比例有了一定的提升，占比由2015年的10%上升至18%。

表7-1 不同检查机构检查药品类型分布情况

检查机构		WHO	EDQM	美国FDA	德国BGV	巴西ANVISA	其他机构	合计
药品类型	原料药	27	12	53	14	10	3	119
	口服固体制剂	14	0	2	1	2	4	23
	注射剂	7	0	2	0	2	8	19
	生物制品	1	0	0	0	4	0	5
	其他	0	0	3	0	0	3	6
	合计	49	12	60	15	18	18	172

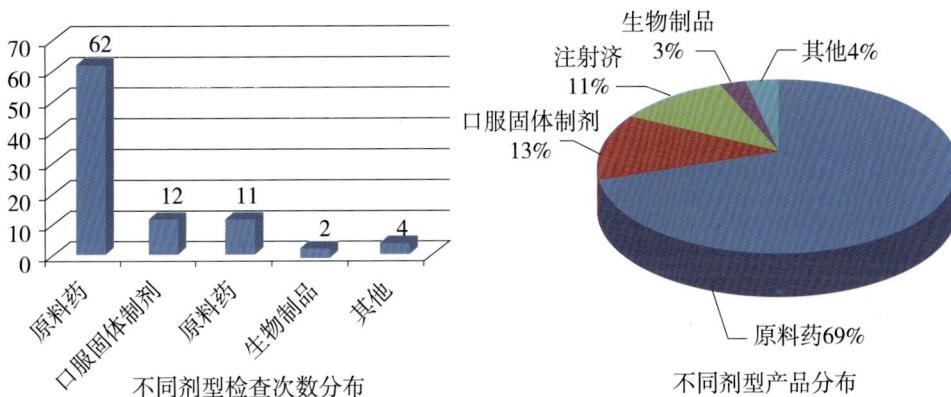

不同剂型检查次数分布

不同剂型产品分布

图7-3 不同机型检查情况分布

二、发现主要问题

2016年观察检查工作中共记录发现的缺陷项1108项，依据我国2010版GMP正文章节对缺陷项进行分类分析发现：质量控制与质量保证、文件管理、设备、物料与产品、确认与验证、厂房与设施六个类别的缺陷占了全部缺陷的88%。与2015年相比，文件管理部分缺陷由第4位上升至第2位，在目前企业逐渐加强数据可靠性管理的环境下仍增长了约7%（由10.5%增加至17.3%），充分体现出当前国外检查对数据可靠性的关注程度与严格要求。

在国外药品GMP检查中，"质量控制与质量保证"部分提出的缺陷占总缺陷数的27.3%，位居首位。主要问题集中在实验室计算机化分析仪器的管理、偏差处理与CAPA、产品质量回顾分析、变更控制、OOS/OOT结果处理、实验室未遵循控制程序的规定、微生物检验管理、质量风险管理、稳定性试验等方面。"文件管理"部分出现的缺陷居于第二位，缺陷主要集中在记录完整性和可追溯性、文件的生命周期管理、文件完整性、记录操作四个方面。"设备"部分出现的缺陷居于第三位，其中设备的使用与清洁、校准、维护与维修、制水系统管理四个方面的缺陷占该部分全部缺陷项的83.6%。"物料与产品"部分的缺陷项集中在供应商管理、物料与产品标识、物料流程管理、物料与产品标准的合规性、放行管理方面。"确认与验证"方面的缺陷主要包括验证的科学性、验证管理、验证文件与记录三类。"厂房与设施"部分的缺陷主要包括环境控制、仓储区管理、降低污染和交叉污染的措施、厂房设施的生命周期管理等四个方面。

三、不同机构药品 GMP 检查分析

检查内容方面，尽管不同药品GMP检查机构检查的重点存在一定的差异，但通过对2016年观察检查中的缺陷情况分析发现：质量控制与质量保证、文件管理、设备、物料与产品、确认与验证、厂房与设施等六个部分出现的缺陷相对较多。在检查最终报告中提出的缺陷条数方面，EDQM、WHO检查出具的缺陷数据相对较多，平均每次检查约20条缺陷，缺陷项目中对检查过程中发现的问题都进行描述，检查结束后整理编写最终检查报告（通常一个月左右）。US FDA在检查中提出的缺陷条数相对较少，平均每次检查约7条缺陷，并不将检查过程中发现的所有问题均作为最终缺陷项，检查员根据发现的问题结合对产品的风险进行判断后形成最终缺陷项，并在召开检查末次会时书面（483表）告知企业。

ANNUAL REPORT OF DRUG INSPECTION 2016

Annual Inspection Report
Series of China Food and Drug
Administration

Written by Center for Food and Drug

Inspection, CFDA

CHINA MEDICAL SCIENCE PRESS

Foreword

The Center for Food and Drug Inspection (CFDI) organized to conduct a total of 431 inspections throughout the year, including pre-approval inspection, GMP certification inspection, GMP follow-up inspection, unannounced inspection, overseas inspection , GSP unannounced inspection and inspection observation.

Overview of the Inspections in 2016

Inspections	Amount of inspected enterprises/ varieties	Amount of inspectorates	Amount of inspectors
Pre-approval inspection	34	43	178
GMP certification inspection	16	16	47
GMP follow-up inspection	204	197	704
Unannounced inspection	39	39	155
Overseas inspection	7	7	31
GSP unannounced inspection	50	50	77
Observation of international inspection	81	81	85
Total	431	433	1277

Contents

Chapter I
Pre-approval Inspection

I. Overview of Inspections

A total of 29 inspection tasks were received in 2016, of which 21 tasks were from the Center for Drug Evaluation of CFDA (hereinafter referred to as CDE), 8 tasks were from the Department of Drug and Cosmetics Registration of CFDA and discipline inspection and supervision departments (for-cause inspection tasks). A total of 178 person-times, 43 inspection teams have been sent out to conduct pre-approval inspection on 34 varieties; 42 on-site inspection reports have been completed, of which 34 passed the inspection, accounting for 81%; and 8 failed or proactively withdrew registration applications, accounting for 19%.

Table 1-1   Information of On-site Inspections

The total number of inspections (varieties)	The number of inspection teams	The number of inspectors
34	43	178

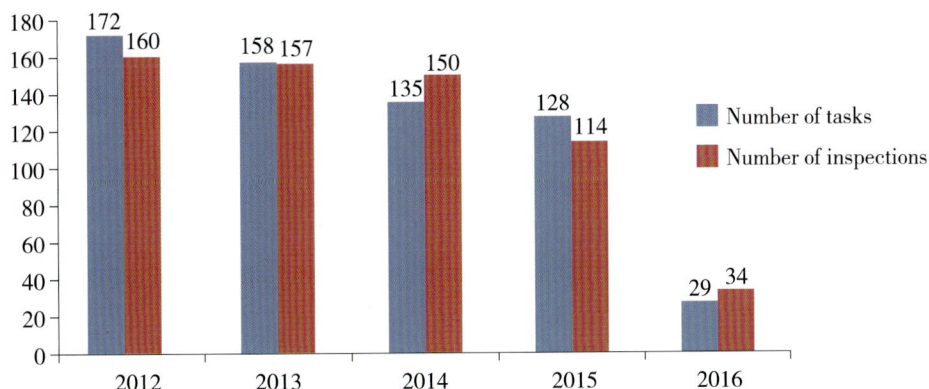

Figure 1-1   Diagram of the Number of Pre-approval Inspection Tasks in Recent Five Years

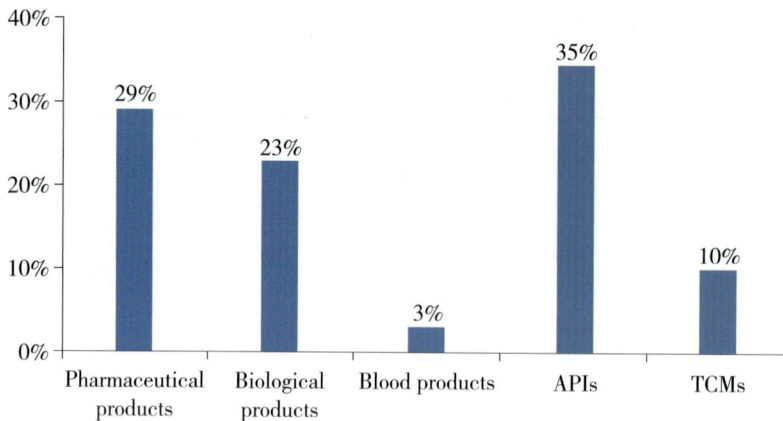

Figure 1-2   Diagram of Dosage Form Distribution in Pre-approval Inspections

II. Main findings

In the pre-approval inspections in 2016, such problems in data integrity as untraceable data and untruthful application dossier were still prominent while insufficient process validation and instable production process and inconsistency between production process or parameters with approved ones were also identified, which were specifically as follows (All issues found in inspection have been dealt in accordance with the law):

(I) Problems in data integrity

(1) Testing data were untraceable. A few enterprises failed to retain samples as required and conduct stability investigation. No retained preproduction samples and retained samples for stability test of the inspected varieties were found in pre-approval inspection, and enterprises also failed to provide both the requisition and destruction records of corresponding retained samples and the samples for stability test and use records of the equipment for stability test.

(2) Batch production records were untruthful and incomplete and inconsistent with application dossier.

(II) The process validation was insufficient and production process was instable

The process validation for the variety was insufficient. During the dynamic production of the enterprises, some procedure had serious deviation or batch product yield had a greater deviation from the validated batch.

(III) The production process or key process parameters and inner packaging materials were inconsistent with the approved ones and no study and assessment was conducted

(1) The production process was inconsistent with that approved / under application.

(2) Key process parameters were inconsistent with the production process approved / under application.

(3) The manufacturer of inner packing materials was inconsistent with that under registration application, and the enterprise did not conduct comparison study.

(IV) Necessary deviation investigation was not conducted

There was significant abnormality in dynamic production, but the investigation was insufficient and the primary cause was not identified. The results of the process validation of three batches and dynamic production batch of the chemical APIs under application by an enterprise showed that there was significant difference in the rate of finished products among four batches, but the enterprise did not analyze and identify the reasons.

Chapter II
Pharmaceutical GMP Certification Inspection

I. Overview of Inspections

Based on the spirit in the Announcement of China Food and Drug Administration on Relevant Issues of Halting the Production by the Enterprises Failing to Pass the Pharmaceutical GMP (revised in 2010) Certification and Decentralizing the Certification of Sterile Pharmaceuticals (2015 No.285), China Food and Drug Administration no longer accepted the application for pharmaceutical GMP certification as of January 1st, 2016. For the certification applications that have been accepted, on-site inspection as well as review and certificate-issuing continued to be completed.

In view of above situation, the inspections on 16 pharmaceutical manufacturers have been arranged, 16 copies of on-site inspection reports have been received and 14 copies have been reviewed throughout the year of 2016. Among them, 12 pharmaceutical manufacturers passed pharmaceutical GMP certification inspection, 2 pharmaceutical manufacturers failed to pass pharmaceutical GMP certification inspection and 5 pharmaceutical manufacturers were issued with Warning Letter; and another two pharmaceutical manufacturers have not yet received approval document for registration so the GMP certification process is suspended.

The dosage forms under application for certification included large volume injection of three enterprises, small volume injection of three enterprises, c of three enterprises, powder injection of one enterprise, radiopharmaceutical of one enterprise, vaccine of two enterprises and other biologics of three enterprises.

Table 2-1　Information of On-site Inspections

The total number of inspections (varieties)	The number of inspection teams	The number of inspectors
16	16	47

Table 2-2   The Distribution of Dosage Forms Subject to Certification Inspection in 2016 (unit: enterprises)

Large volume injection	Small volume injection	Freeze-dried powder injection	Powder injection	Radio-pharmaceutical	Vaccine	Biologics (others)
3	3	3	1	1	2	3

II. Main findings

A total of 220 deficiencies were identified, including 23 major deficiencies and 197 general deficiencies. There were 41 deficiencies in Quality Control and Quality Assurance, 32 deficiencies in Documentation Management, 24 deficiencies in Institutions and Personnel, 23 deficiencies in Equipment and 21 deficiencies in Verification and Qualification. The distribution was basically consistent with that in 2015.

The two manufacturers of in vitro diagnostic reagents receiving certification inspection all failed this year. The main problems were as follows:

(I) Quality Management System

Quality management system could not be effective operated and failed to meet the production and quality requirements of the products; The personnel mobility was frequent, there lacked professionals and the training was not conducted, which could not meet the quality management requirements in routine production; The operability of the documents were poor and data were incompletely recorded; relevant changes were not subject to change control in accordance with change procedure.

(II) Verification and Qualification

The enterprises failed to conduct process validation for all the products under application for GMP certification, and the cleaning validation for public equipment and facilities was not in place; part of validation records was incomplete; and some re-validation work was not conducted as required.

Chapter III
Pharmaceutical GMP
Follow-up Inspection

I. Overview of Inspections

In 2016, it was planned in the Announcement to conduct follow-up inspection on 215 enterprises, a total of 228 inspections. Among them, 58 inspections were conducted on the enterprises out of production or having no production for a long time, and other 170 inspections have all been conducted.

In addition, follow-up inspection was conducted on 21 sterile drug manufacturers passing provincial certification, and double random inspection was conducted on 13 enterprises. A total of 204 follow-up inspections were completed.

Table 3-1   Information of GMP Follow-up Inspections

The total number of inspections (manufacturers)	The number of inspection teams	The number of inspectors
204	197	704

Table 3-2   Information of Inspection Distribution

Categories	Amount of planned inspections	Amount of actual inspections
The enterprises unqualified in casual inspection in 2015	11	10
The enterprises issued with Warning Letter in 2015	37	32
Vaccine manufacturers	38	36
Blood product manufacturers	28	25
Manufacturers of high-risk varieties	114	67

continue table

Categories	Amount of planned inspections	Amount of actual inspections
Sterile drug manufacturers passing provincial certification	21	21
Double random inspection	13	13
Total	262	204

12 enterprises failed in follow-up inspection, accounting for 5.9%, and 58 enterprises were issued with Warning Letter, accounting for 28.9%.

Among 12 enterprises failing in the inspection, there were 5 enterprises unqualified in casual inspection in 2015, 4 enterprises subject to double random inspection, 2 manufacturers of citicoline sodium injection and 1 manufacturer of ossotide injection (All issues found in inspection have been dealt in accordance with the law).

(I) The situation of casual inspection of the varieties in quality report in 2015

10 enterprises accepted the follow-up inspection on such dosage forms and varieties as eye drops, bendazol tablets and APIs of sodium benzoate, of which 5 enterprises failed, accounting for 50%, and 4 enterprises were issued with Warning Letter.

(II) Double random inspection

In order to implement the requirements of innovating the supervision inwards and afterwards by the State Council, in accordance with the unified arrangement by CFDA, double random inspection system for pharmaceuticals was initially operated in December 2016, follow-up inspection was conducted on the 13 selected enterprises. The inspections distributed in 9 provinces and involved 3 chemicals, 2 APIs and 8 TCMs. 4 enterprises failed in the inspection, and the pass rate was only 69%. In addition, 3 enterprises were issued with Warning Letter.

(III) Vaccine manufacturers

38 vaccine manufacturers that have obtained GMP certificate were marketed in the follow-up inspection plan in 2016. Except for 1 enterprise having production license and GMP certificate revoked in 2014 and 1 enterprise failing to get GMP certification in 2015 due to the application for the change of production address, the follow-up inspection was conducted on other 36 vaccine manufacturers. All 36 enterprises passed the inspection, and 7 enterprises which found general risks and can be improved by rectification were issued with Warning

Letter. According to experts assessment that one critical deficiency that was evaluated by inspectors on site should be decreased to major deficiency, being low risk. On the whole, the quality risks in vaccine production are controllable and the manufacturers have a standardized production and quality management.

(IV) Blood product manufacturers

26 blood product manufacturers were marketed in the follow-up inspection plan in 2016. Except for 1 enterprise in production suspension and rectification, the follow-up inspection was conducted on other 25 blood product manufacturers. All 25 enterprises passed the inspection, and 4 enterprises which found general risks and can be improved by rectification were issued with Warning Letter. On the whole, the quality risks in blood product production are controllable, the manufacturers have a standardized production and quality management, but the supervision shall be intensified for individual enterprises.

(V) The manufacturers issued with warning letter in 2015

Follow-up inspection has been conducted on 32 manufacturers issued with warning letter in 2015. The manufacturers were basically met the requirements, but 14 manufacturers were issued with warning letter again.

(VI) The situation of casual inspections on the sterile drug manufacturers passing provincial certification after the decentralization of certification

21 sterile drug manufacturers passing provincial certification received casual inspection. All of them passed the inspection and 6 enterprises were issued with Warning Letter. According to the inspection result, the Provincial Bureau can undertake the GMP certification inspection functions smoothly down.

(VII) Special inspection on high-risk varieties

This year, follow-up inspection was mainly conducted on the injection of three products including ossotide, fructose diphosphate and citicoline sodium. It was planned to conduct 114 special inspections on high-risk varieties. 47 enterprises were not inspected because of failing in GMP (2010 version) certification, out of production for a long time and transfer of approval number, and 67 inspections were actually conducted. In the inspections, 1 ossotide injection manufacturer and 2 citicoline sodium injection manufacturers failed, and 21 manufacturers were issued with Warning Letter.

II. Main findings

(I) Overall situation

A total of 2271 deficiencies were identified in 204 inspections, of which there were 22 critical deficiencies, 210 major deficiencies and 2039 general deficiencies. Compared with GMP certification and follow-up inspections in 2015, the number of critical deficiencies was increased.

Among the manufacturers of high-risk varieties subject to special inspection, out of production for a long time or failing in pharmaceutical GMP (2010 version) certification were prominent. The common problems identified in the inspections were as follows:

(1) Individual enterprise had inconsistency between its production process and registered process.

(2) The problems in data integrity and authenticity still existed, including falsification of production records, indiscriminate use of maps and arbitrary modification of data in inspection records and inconsistency in relevant content in production, equipment and material records.

(3) The process validation was insufficient, and the enterprises failing to conduct process validation after changing production lot size had more problems.

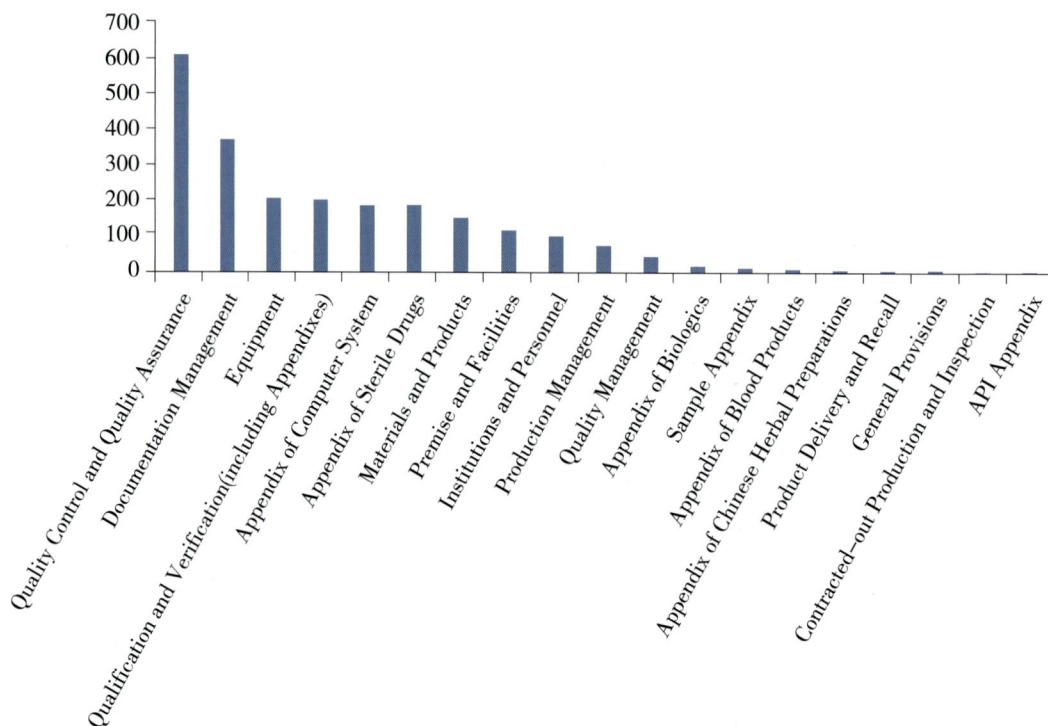

Figure 3-1 Distribution of the Deficiencies Identified in Follow-up Inspections

(4) The problems in the standardization of data management were prominent, mainly manifesting as failing to control the permission setting of the system, audit tracking function and the permission for the modification and deletion of documents and data, and having no reasonable control and explanation for deleting, selecting and using data.

(5) There was certain gap between the implementation of the Appendix of Computer System and Appendix of Qualification and Validation and regulatory requirements, and many problems were identified.

(6) There was a weak management of deviations and changes, mainly manifesting as failing to effectively identify and record the deviations that occurred, and lacking necessary assessment and validation for the changes.

(II) The enterprises unqualified in casual inspections in 2015

A total of 11 critical deficiencies, 27 major deficiencies and 84 general deficiencies were identified in the inspections on 11 enterprises.

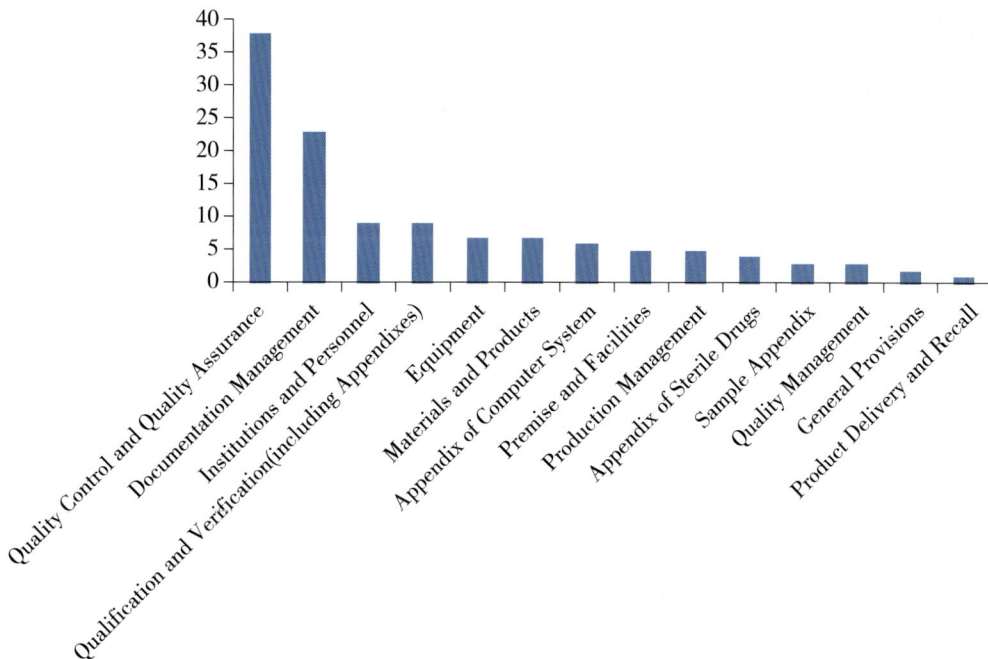

Figure 3-2   Distribution of the Deficiencies of the Enterprises Unqualified in Casual Inspection

Main findings were as follows:

(1) Production process was inconsistent with registered process.

(2) Problems in data integrity.

(3) Problems in process validation.

(III) Double random inspection

A total of 5 critical deficiencies, 24 major deficiencies and 123 general deficiencies were identified.

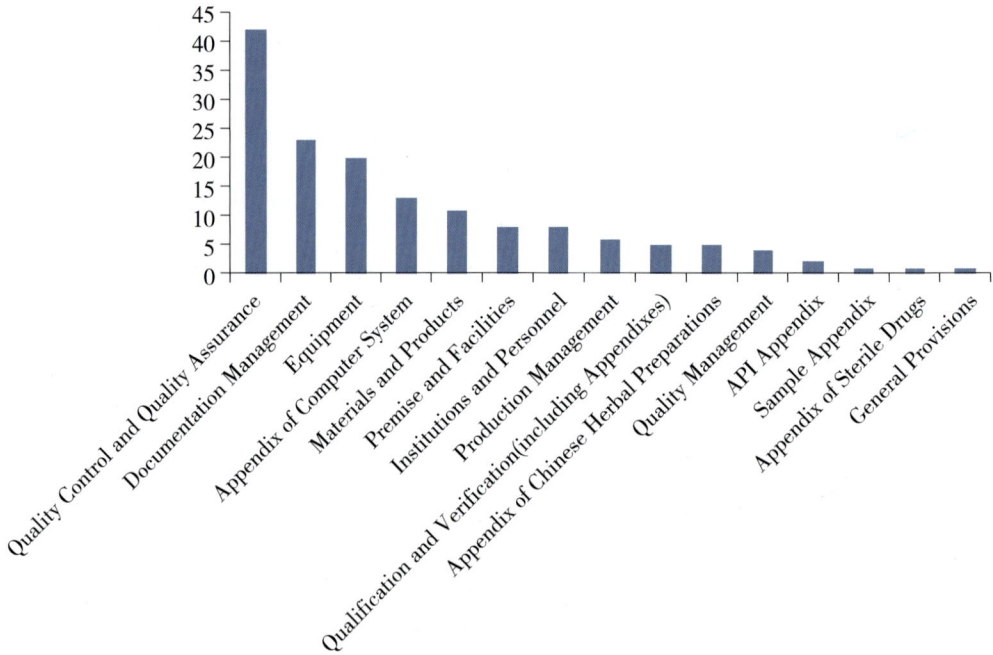

Figure 3-3   Distribution of the Deficiencies Identified in Double Random Inspections

Main findings were as follows:

(1) Record falsification.

(2) Potential hazards in product quality and safety.

(3) Problems in data integrity.

(4) Problems in process validation.

(5) Non-standardized material management with the risks in pollution, confusion and error.

(6) Incomplete cleaning, which cannot effectively prevent contamination and cross-contamination.

(IV) Vaccine manufacturers

38 major deficiencies and 383 general deficiencies were identified.

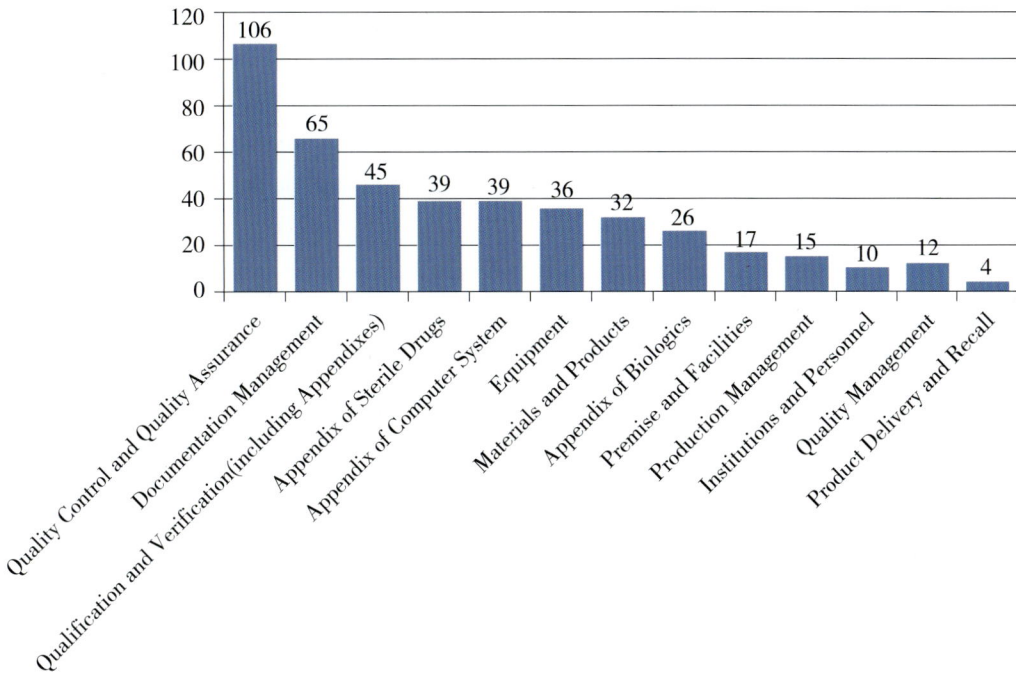

Figure 3-4   Distribution of the Deficiencies of Vaccine Manufacturers identified in the inspections

Main findings:

1. Equipment

There was a too long stagnant water section between the stainless steel pipe valve through which water for injection preparation system enters into injection water storage tank and water generator; Individual device had rust.

2. Materials and Products

The quantity of the destructed items was not recorded in the destruction records of the non-conforming finished products; the enterprise failed to establish the background information of whole genome sequence of main bacterial and viral seeds for production.

3. Documentation Management

Individual document was not specifically specified and was poor in its operability. The content specified in the document was inconsistent with the actual situation; individual record had incomplete content; the batch production records were unreasonably designed and were not timely filled in actual operation.

4. Quality Control and Quality Assurance

(1) Quality management of laboratories: the enterprise failed to request necessary test data and maps from the institutions conducting entrusted test; some material was subject to infrared

test after sample mixing.

(2) the Deviation handling: The training and implementation of the documents related to deviation handling was not conducted; the enterprise failed to timely initiate the investigation for individual deviation; the reason analysis and corrective and preventive measures for a few deviations were not in place, and there was in adequate assessment on the potential impact of the deviations on the quality of products.

(3) Change control: The enterprise failed to handle the changes in accordance with change process and submit supplementary application for registration. There was no or inadequate assessment on some changes;

(4) Supplier management: There was incomplete auditing content for the suppliers of some materials, and the enterprise failed to determine the auditing content for suppliers based on the impact of the material on product quality.

(5) Product quality review: The enterprise failed to conduct annual quality review by varieties.

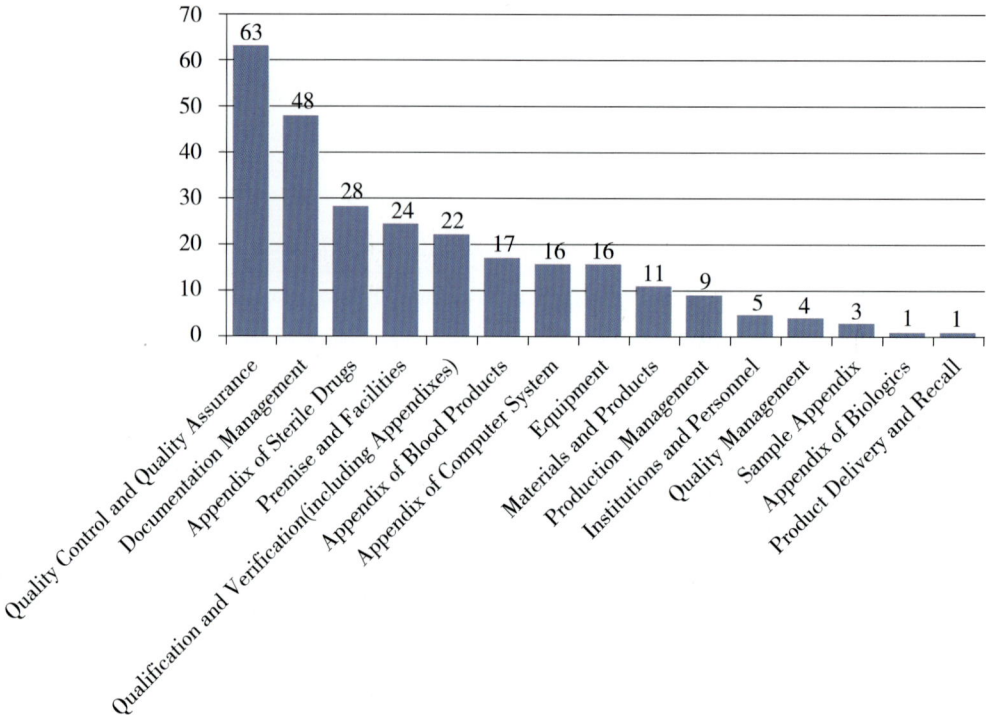

Figure 3-5   Distribution of the Deficiencies of Blood Product Manufacturers Identified in the Inspections

5. Computer System

The enterprise has developed document system for computer system management, but did not conduct classification management in accordance with the system, and did not take effective measures to reduce risks for the situation that existing conditions failed to comply with the document; there was no permission setting for the login screen of HPLC testing equipment in quality verification laboratory, and no measures to prevent the login by the unauthorized person.

(V) Blood product manufacturers

In the inspections on 25 enterprises, 13 major deficiencies and 241 general deficiencies were identified, and no critical deficiency was identified.

Main findings:

1. Institutions and Personnel

There lacked training for the personnel at some posts.

2. Premises and Facilities

The contamination and cross contamination cannot be effectively controlled.

3. Equipment

Some sensors failed to cover the actual use range; some instruments and equipment for testing were not regularly calibrated or insufficiently calibrated, and the records were incomplete; the equipment had no status identification and calibration identification.

4. Materials and Products

There lacked the source, validity period and other information on the label of the cryo in allocated supply, and the label was a card, which was easy to be lost and confused.

5. Verification and Qualification

In simulated filling test of culture media, sampling monitoring was conducted for both hands, forearms and chest of operators only after the production was over, and the sampling of clothes as well as the confirmation was not specified.

6. Documentation Management

The technological procedure and operating procedure was not specific in content, poor in operability and not standardized in the provisions..

7. Production Management

There lacked microbial control measures for the octylic acid sodium solution added before inactivation; The time to place the settlement plate under Level A laminar flow was not confirmed.

8. Quality Control and Quality Assurance

(1) Management of quality control laboratories: the machine account for the receiving and

dispatching of tested products had incomplete content, and there was no receiving information of the test samples of intermediates and semi-finished products; the plate culture medium outsourced for environmental monitoring was not tested; negative control was not set for sterility test in accordance with the pharmacopoeia;

(2) Product stability study: Invalidity period was formulated for intermediate products, but there lacked the support of continuous stability investigation or validation data;

(3) Change control: Change control and management was not in place. Some changes were not or insufficiently assessed;

(4) Deviation handling: the enterprise failed to timely initiate the investigation for individual deviation; some deviation investigation and corrective and preventive measures were insufficient;

(5) Supplier management: The allocated suppliers of cryo was not included in the directory of qualified suppliers of the enterprise;

(6) Product quality review: Some information was not included in annual product quality review;

(7) Product delivery and recall: The enterprise failed to specify the shipment means for the sample in batch release;

(8) Computer System: there were incomplete documents for computer system, and there lacked comprehensive and effective control and assessment for internal computer system and relevant data. There was no auditing and tracking function for some instruments and equipment in QC laboratory; the system did not set access permission at different levels, and there was a risk of data and system modification; the safety and reliability of HPLC data transfer was not confirmed.

(VI) The manufacturers issued with Warning Letter in 2015

For the inspections on 32 manufacturers, a total of 2 critical deficiencies, 32 major deficiencies and 328 general deficiencies were identified.

Main findings were as follows:

(1) Problems in data integrity.

(2) No records and investigations for the deviations.

(3) There were certain problems in sterility guarantee and relevant verification and qualification work was inadequate.

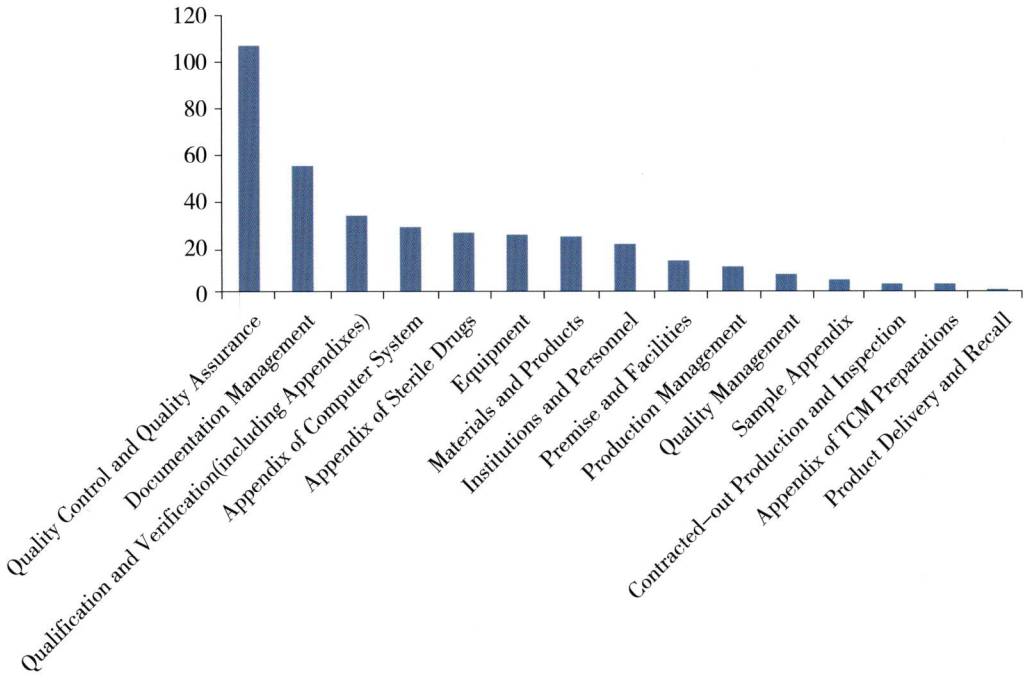

Figure 3-6   Distribution of the Deficiencies of the Enterprises Issued with Warning Letter Identified in the Inspections in 2015

(VII) The Sterile Drug Manufacturers Passing Provincial Certification

In the inspections on 21 enterprises, a total of 15 major deficiencies and 209 general deficiencies were identified, but no critical deficiency was identified.

The main problems identified manifested as: there is insufficient risk assessment for sharing production line in the production of small volume injection; there was cleaning validation for single variety, but no cleaning risk assessment for all the varieties; some inspection records had incomplete content; the validation and audit of computer system has not yet been carried out; materials were improperly managed, and there were risks of confusion and error.

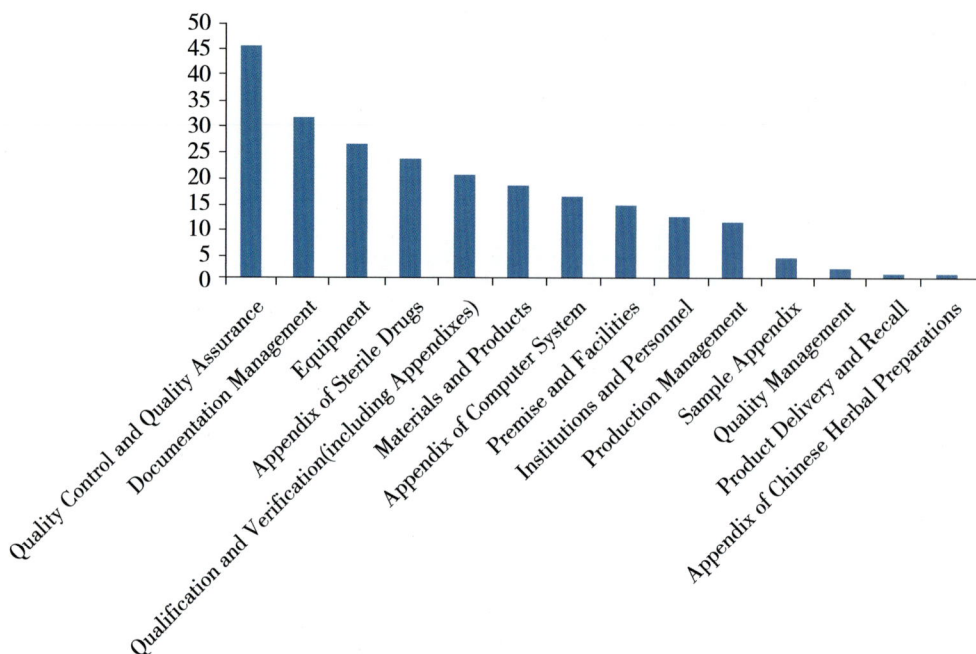

Figure 3-7   Distribution of the Deficiencies of the Sterile Drug Manufacturers Passing Provincial Certification in Follow-up Inspections

(VIII) Special inspections on high-risk varieties

In the inspections on 61 enterprises, a total of 3 critical deficiencies, 64 major deficiencies and 658 general deficiencies were identified.

Main findings were as follows:

1. Ossotide injection

(1) The company bought 7 batches of foreleg bone from XX Co. Ltd., but failed to conduct procurement and acceptance inspection according to stipulations. The company failed to formulate procurement order according to procurement SOP. After the arrival of materials, the company failed to request and check the inspection report issued by the supplier in accordance with the SOP for the acceptance inspection, warehousing and storage of materials; for the acceptance inspection, the company failed to request temperature monitoring record of cold chain transportation of pig legs.

(2) The virus inactivation for the stock solution of compound ossotide was not validated; there was validation data to support that the four pig legs shall be stored for 25 days after requisition and the time from filling to sterilization initiation of compound ossotide injection is five hours; the time from the end of preparation to the end of the filling of compound ossotide

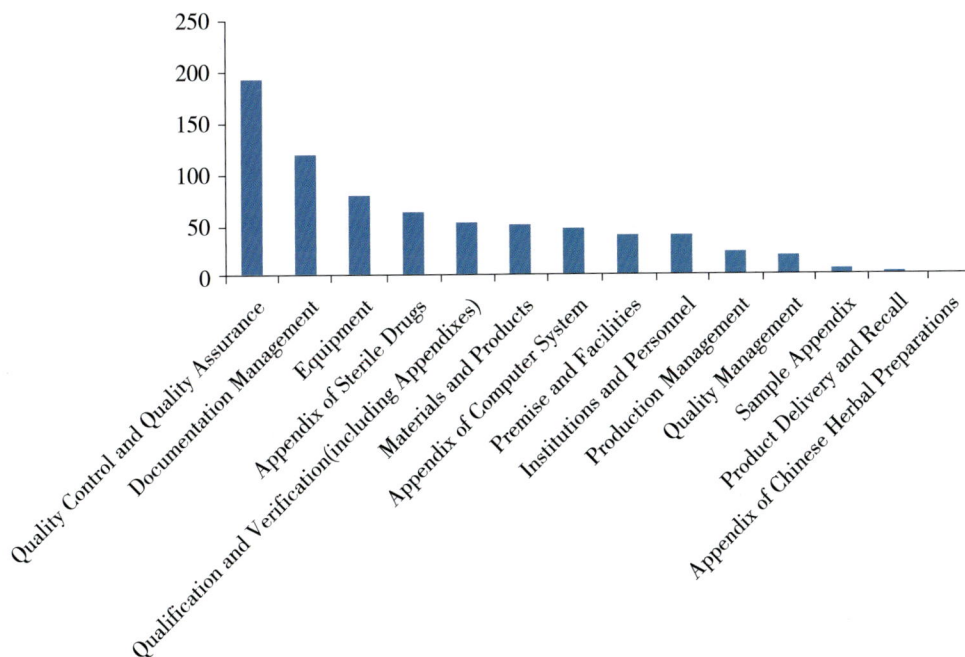

Figure 3-8   Distribution of the Deficiencies of High-risk Varieties Identified in Special Inspection

injection was 10 hours, which lacked the microbial limit detection data.

(3) The continuous stability test scheme failed to set and inspect such activity indicators and related safety indicators as allergic experiment, pyrogen, and abnormal toxicity.

2. Fructose diphosphate injection

(1) The criteria for microbial limit in internal control standard of fructose diphosphate manufacturers failed to be revised in accordance with corresponding provisions in Chinese pharmacopoeia (2015 edition).

(2) For the compound enzyme reagent used for the content determination of the APIs of fructose diphosphate, the expiration date was December 2015. It was found in on-site inspection that the enterprise still used such enzyme reagent to conduct content determination of 14 batches of APIs of fructose diphosphate after the expiration date.

3. Citicoline sodium injection

(1) The inner quality standard for the APIs of citicoline sodium was unreasonably developed, and the item of toluene residue was not added with reference to the quality standard of APIs manufacturers.

(2) For the comparison of the content determination methods of intermediates and finished products of citicoline sodium injection, it was conducted only for the detection result of one

batch and was not representative.

(3) The enterprise of citicoline sodium injection failed to conduct process validation for the APIs of different manufacturers respectively; the enterprise failed to provide compatibility test data of sterilizing filter for citicoline sodium injection.

Chapter IV
Unannounced Inspection for Pharmaceuticals

I. Overview of Inspection

In accordance with the requirements for relevant departments of CFDA, based on the Working Procedure for Unannounced Inspection on Pharmaceutical GMP, a total of 45 unannounced inspection tasks from CFDA have been received in 2016, of which 39 unannounced inspections on Pharmaceutical GMP have been completed with the results reported, and others are on-going. The 39 inspections with the results reported involved 20 provinces (municipalities) including Beijing, Jiangsu and Guangdong etc., and covered 9 manufacturers of biochemical drugs, 20 manufacturers of TCMs, 9 manufacturers of chemicals and 1 manufacturer of blood product. The distribution was as follows:

Of the unannounced inspection tasks in 2016, 33 tasks were from the Department of Drug and Cosmetics Supervision of CFDA, and 6 tasks were from the Department of Drug and Cosmetics Registration and other departments of CFDA. The tasks from the Department of Drug and Cosmetics Supervision of CFDA accounted for 85%, which was the main source of unannounced inspection tasks. Among 39 unannounced inspections, the inspections on TCMs accounted for 51% of all the unannounced inspection work while that on chemicals and biochemical drugs accounted for 23%, respectively. In the unannounced inspection in 2016, 21 drug manufacturers failed, accounting for 54%. It was suggested to revoke the pharmaceutical GMP certificate of 14 enterprises and to open an investigation for 10 enterprises. The problematic products of 7 enterprises were ordered to be recalled. In pharmaceutical GMP unannounced inspection, TCMs and chemical drugs were identified to have more problems. All issues found in unannounced inspection have been dealt in accordance with the law.

Table 4-1   Handling of unannounced inspections

Product category	Amount of inspections	Fail	Revocation of GMP certificate	Product recall
TCMs	20	14	9	2
Biochemical drugs	9	5	4	4
Blood products	1	1	1	1
Chemicals	9	1	0	0

II. Main findings

(I) Main problems identified in TCMs manufacturers

In 2016, a total of 66 person-times in 18 teams of inspectorates were sent for unannounced inspections on 20 TCMs manufacturers, of which there were 6 manufacturers involving letter reporting, there were 3 manufacturers of calculus bovis factitious, 7 manufacturers of the products containing bezoar, 3 enterprises identified to have problems in exploration study and inspection and 1 manufacturer of prepared slices of Chinese crude medicines.

In the unannounced inspection on 20 TCMs manufacturers, 12 manufacturers failed to meet pharmaceutical GMP requirements, of which three manufacturers were transferred to provincial administration for handling relevant problems, one manufacturer was issued with Warning Letter, one manufacturer had no relevant production and three manufacturers met the requirements.

1. Chinese patent medicine manufacturers

(1) The problem of unauthorized changes to the process was prominent.

In order to reduce the production cost of oral preparation of Chinese patent medicine, the phenomenon of unauthorized changes to the pretreatment and extraction process is still a prominent problem. The unannounced inspections conducted this year were due to the problems identified in exploratory inspection, such as the enterprise failed to extract some Chinese herbal medicine in the prescription that should be extracted in accordance with technological procedure, but conducted a direct feeding after smashing.

(2) The Chinese herbal medicine and prepared slices of Chinese crude medicines was in disordered management.

In order to cope with the supervisory inspection by the drug regulatory authorities at all levels, individual manufacturer of Chinese patent medicine falsified machine account of warehouse materials and stock in and stock out record. The relevant machine account and records of the materials for internal operation in such enterprises can correspond to each other, but failed to respond to the invoice or voucher for the purchase. Or, such enterprises took advantage of such policy that the Chinese herbal medicine can be purchased directly from farmers, reversely inferred the usage of Chinese herbal medicine from the production of Chinese patent medicine, and then fabricated the machine account of materials according to the demand.

(3) The purchased Chinese herbal medicine and prepared slices of Chinese crude medicines were not subject to strict full inspection and the data integrity was doubtable.

Traditional manufacturers of Chinese patent medicine have many varieties of products and involve may varieties of Chinese herbal medicine and prepared slices of Chinese crude medicines. Because the precision analysis instruments and QC personnel equipped were not adapted to the scale of production, it cannot be ensured that each batch of the purchased Chinese herbal medicine and prepared slices of Chinese crude medicines can be inspected, resulting in no full inspection for the Chinese herbal medicine and prepared slices of Chinese crude medicines of some batch, or using a graph for multi-purpose to deal with the inspection.

2. Calculus bovis factitius

Because calculus bovis factitious is marketed under the classification of "Medicinal Materials and Prepared Slices" in the Chinese pharmacopoeia, it belongs to raw materials for Chinese patent medicine, resulting in that relevant enterprises cannot organize the production in accordance with pharmaceutical GMP requirements. In particular, there were seriously insufficient requirements for the auditing and management of the suppliers of upstream industry chain of calculus bovis factitious, causing that hygienic conditions of processing site were bad, the raw materials could not be traced and the processing process was uncontrollable. Main fingings:

(1) The management of suppliers was weak.

(2) The authenticity of microbial limit test was doubtful.

(3) It failed to be included in quality assurance system.

3. Prepared slices of Chinese crude medicines

A variety of information showed that the dispensing for sales was very common for the prepared slices of Chinese crude medicines outsourced. The problems in content determination of purchased Chinese herbal medicines or process products were prominent, dyeing and weight increment problems occurred occasionally, and authenticity of batch production records was doubtful.

(1) Untruthful batch production records.

(2) Being suspected of dispensing and sale of outsourcing prepared slices.

(3) Authenticity problems in data integrity.

(II) Biochemical drugs

1. Inspection on " monosialotetrahexosylganglioside sodium"

In 2016, a total of 4 manufacturers of " monosialotetrahexosylganglioside sodium" were inspected, and it was found that there was certain risk in the management of the quality of raw materials and the pig brain suppliers.

(1) Supplier management shall be improved, for the management of suppliers by the enterprise cannot ensure effective traceability.

(2) There was insufficient management of electronic data of the monitoring of cold chain transport of pig brain.

2. Inspection on " hepatocyte growth-promoting factors for injection"

In 2016, a total of 4 manufacturers of " hepatocyte growth-promoting factors for injection" were inspected, of which 2 manufacturers had their Pharmaceutical GMP Certificate revoked while 2 manufacturers were issued with Warning Letter.

(1) Fabricate the record file.

(2) Problems in data integrity

(3) Inconsistency with registered production process

(4) Unable to effectively ensure the quality of the liver as raw material.

Chapter V
Overseas Inspections for
Imported Pharmaceuticals

I. Overview of Inspections

(I) Overview of annual inspection tasks

The total number of CFDA Overseas Inspection was 49 inspections.

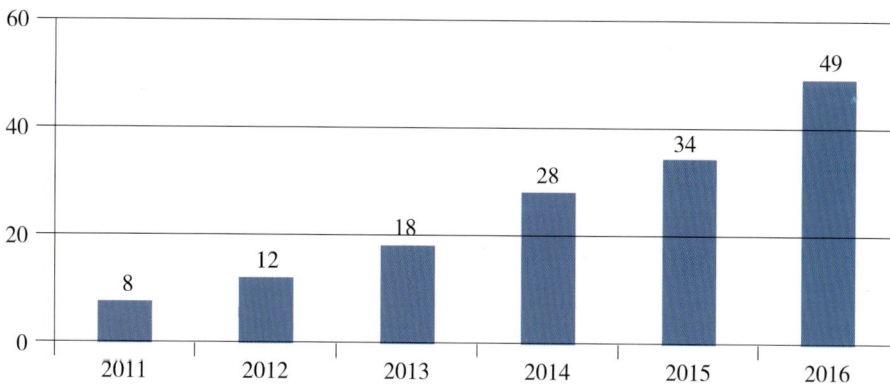

Figure 5-1   Amount of Overseas Inspection Tasks in 2011-2016

(1) The inspection tasks in 2016 involved 19 countries. There were relatively more varieties in Europe and North America, the varieties of such countries with high regional quality risks as India and Vietnam account for certain proportion, and at the same time, the inspection on the varieties in South America and Australia was also intensified.

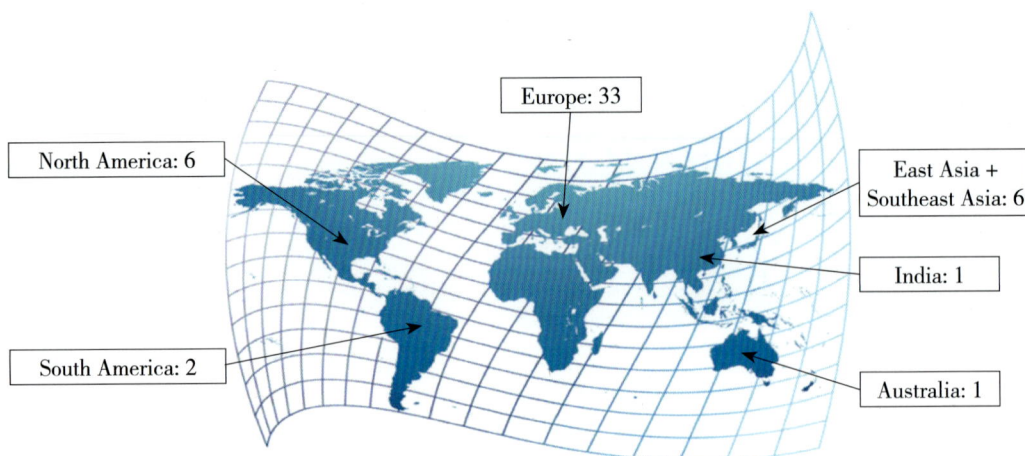

Figure 5-2   Country Distribution of Planned Inspection Tasks in 2016

(2) The inspection followed the principle that inspection shall serve the evaluation and approval and took into consideration the safety requirements for the marketed products. The proportion of the varieties under review was increased, and the product under application for clinical trials, application for production and re-registration and in the stage of supplementary application shall all be included in the scope of inspection. The reason for the inspection on the marketed products was mainly port quality inspection problems. The iodoprestamine injection, a variety with high risks in adverse reaction monitoring manufactured by a foreign company, was added for inspection.

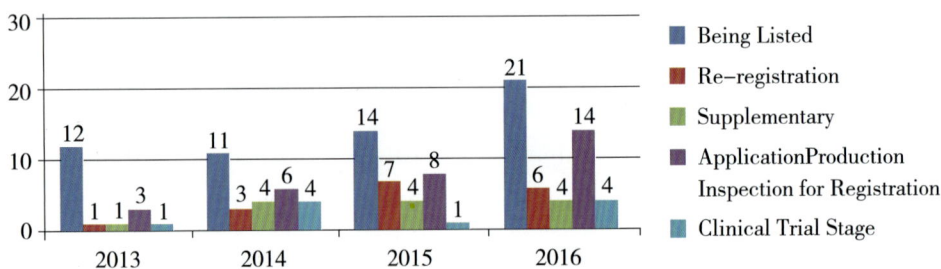

Figure 5-3   Registration Status of Inspection Tasks in Recent Years

(3) The inspection tasks were characterized as comprehensive varieties and broad dosage forms, and the extended inspection on chemical preparations was intensified. 40 chemicals were involved, including injections, solid preparations, implant and nasal sprays, of which there were 3 biochemical products, 6 APIs for extended inspection; 11 vaccines, blood products and therapeutic biological products; and 4 botanical drugs.

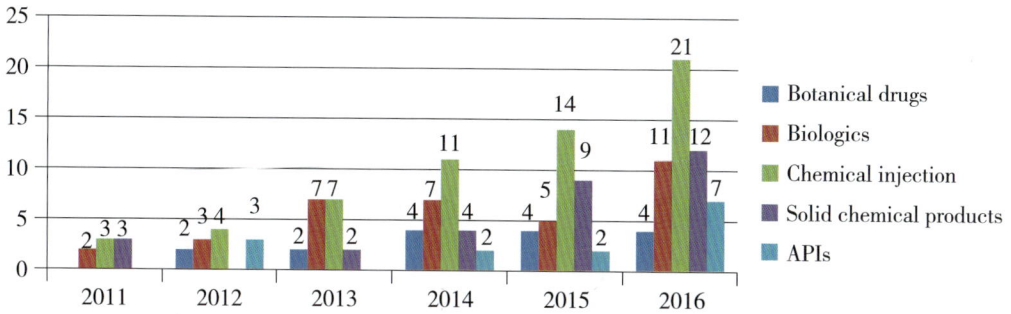

Figure 5-4   Classification of Inspection Tasks

(II) The implementation of the inspections in 2016

Due to the inspection tour of CFDA and CFDI in the first half year, the change in relevant foreign affairs and production arrangement of enterprises, CFDI submit the inspection tasks of 37 varieties throughout the year: the inspection tasks of 15 varieties have been completed, of which on-site inspection was conducted on 7 varieties, and three of them failed, accounting for 42%; the enterprises of 8 varieties proactively withdrew the import registration certificate or had their application returned during the organization of the inspections, account for 17% of total annual plan. For another 21 varieties, due to production scheduling of enterprises, the inspection is scheduled to be completed in the first quarter of 2017, and relevant formalities of foreign affairs are being dealt with. For the other 12 varieties, because the enterprises cannot accept inspection in the first quarter of 2017, CFDI has reported to the Department of Drug and Cosmetics Supervision to include them in the overseas inspections in 2017.

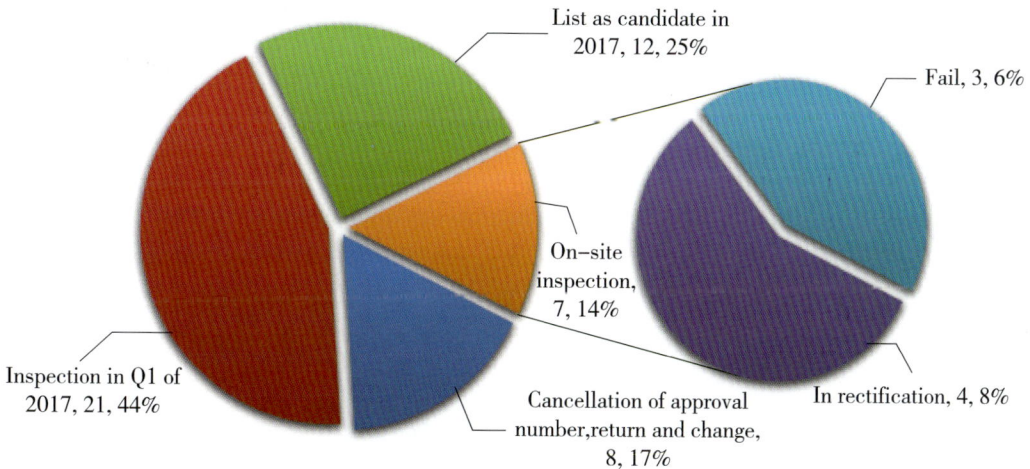

Figure 5-5   The Situation of the Inspections in 2016

II. Main findings in overseas inspections

Among 7 varieties that have been inspected, three varieties failed, and the failure rate was slightly increased compared with previous years. 117 deficiencies have been identified in the inspections, of which there were 3 critical deficiencies and 18major deficiencies. The problems mainly focused on Quality Control and Quality Assurance, Material System and Change Management; and critical deficiencies were mainly the problems in the consistency of production process and data integrity. All issues found in overseas inspection have been dealt in accordance with the law.

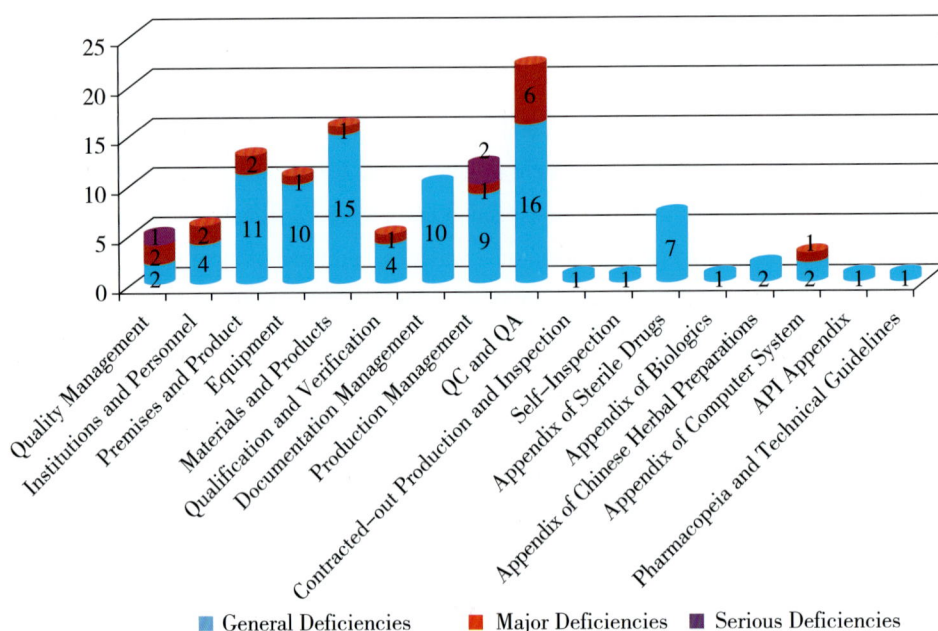

Figure 5-6   Summarization and Analysis of the Deficiencies Identified in the Overseas Inspections in 2016

Main and serious problems were as follows:

(1) Actual production process and production site was inconsistent with those in registration application and major changes were implemented without submitting application in China.

(2) There were significant problems in data integrity, which serious affected the product quality.

(3) There were an increasing number of varieties handled by off-site inspection.

Chapter VI
GSP unannounced inspection

I. Overview of Inspections

In 2016, China Food and Drug Administration conducted centralized remediation on illegal distribution behaviors in drug circulation field, further reorganized and regulated drug circulation order through self-inspection and rectification by enterprises, supervision and inspection by provincial administration and unannounced inspection by CFDA and cracked down illegal distribution behaviors. Throughout the year, 3 batches of inspections have been conducted on 53 pharmaceutical wholesalers. The results of unannounced inspections were announced by CFDA.

Table 6-1　Information of annual tasks of pharmaceutical circulation inspection in 2016

Batch of unannounced inspection	Amount of inspected enterprises	Amount of inspects (person-time)
The first batch	28	37
The second batch	11	20
The third batch	11	20
Total	50	77

The teams of inspectorates conducted unannounced inspection on relevant enterprises based on the Announcement of CFDA on Remediating Illegal Distribution Behaviors in Drug Circulation Field (2016 No.94) and Good Supply Practice for Pharmaceuticals. It was identified in the results that the violations were very common in drug circulation enterprises, and the situation was as follows.

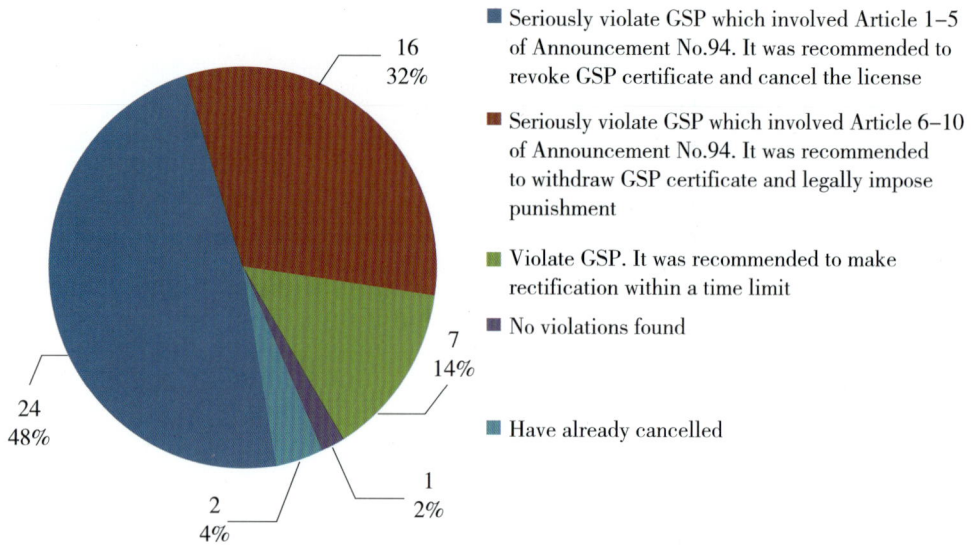

- Seriously violate GSP which involved Article 1–5 of Announcement No.94. It was recommended to revoke GSP certificate and cancel the license
- Seriously violate GSP which involved Article 6–10 of Announcement No.94. It was recommended to withdraw GSP certificate and legally impose punishment
- Violate GSP. It was recommended to make rectification within a time limit
- No violations found
- Have already cancelled

Figure 6-1 Results of unannounced inspection on 53 pharmaceutical wholesalers

II. Main findings

(I) The situation of violations of CFDA Announcement No.94

Table 6-2 The situation of violations of CFDA Announcement No.94 by enterprises identified in unannounced inspection in drug circulation enterprises

Relevant clauses in Announcement No.94	The number of suspected manufacturers	Proportion
(I) Provide a site, qualification certificate, bills and other conditions for illegal distribution of drugs by others	10	20%
(II) Purchase drugs from individuals or a unit without Pharmaceutical Production License and Pharmaceutical Distribution License	1	2%
(III) Sell drugs to a unit without legal qualification or individuals, sell vaccines to drug retailers, or provide drugs to others under the situation that one knows or shall know others are engaged in unlicensed business activities	1	2%
(IV) Falsify the source for drug procurement, fabricate sales flow of drugs, tamper the data of computer system and temperature and humidity monitoring system, conceal the real drug purchase-sales-storage records, bills, voucher and data, the drug purchase-sales-storage records are incomplete and untruthful and distribution behaviors are untraceable	16	32%

continue table

Relevant clauses in Announcement No.94	The number of suspected manufacturers	Proportion
(V) For purchase and sales of drugs, the certificate (license certificate), bills (invoice, the sheet along with the goods), account (materials account, financial account), goods (drugs) and money (payment for drugs) cannot be corresponding to or consistent with each other; fail to warehouse the drugs with concealed accounts established, fail to manage the drugs after including them into quality management system, use personal account to conduct business dealings, and other situations	19	38%
(VI) Make the narcotic drugs, psychotropic substances and compound preparations containing special drugs flow into illegal channel or conduct cash transaction	3	6%
(VII) Store the drugs outside of the approved addressed	6	12%
(VIII) Fail to store and transport the drugs and monitor the temperature and humidity in accordance with the regulations	21	42%
(IX) Arbitrarily change registration address, business patter and business scope to sell drugs	5	10%
(X) Fail to issue a sales invoice and ensure its being along with the drugs when selling drugs to drug retailers and clinics	6	12%

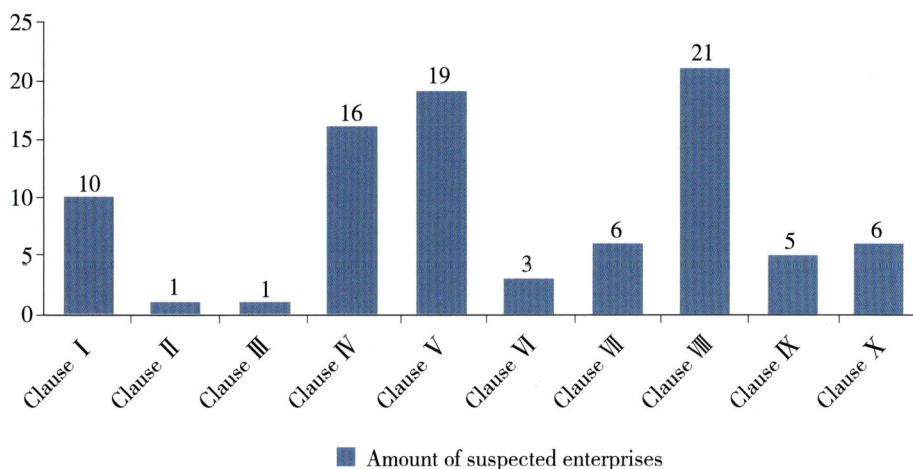

Figure 6-2   Distribution of the Clauses in Announcement No.94 Violated by Enterprises

Main findings:

(1) Fail to store and transport the drugs and monitor the temperature and humidity in accordance with the regulations.

(2) For purchase and sales of drugs, the certificate (license certificate), bills (invoice, the sheet along with the goods), account (materials account, financial account), goods (drugs) and money (payment for drugs) cannot be corresponding to or consistent with each other; fail to warehouse the drugs with concealed accounts established, fail to manage the drugs after including them into quality management system, use personal account to conduct business dealings, and other situations.

(3) The enterprises falsified the source for drug procurement, fabricated sales flow of drugs, tampered the data of computer system and temperature and humidity monitoring system, and concealed the real drug purchase-sales-storage records, bills, voucher and data, the drug purchase-sales-storage records were incomplete and untruthful and distribution behaviors were untraceable.

(II) The situation of violation of Good Supply Practice for Pharmaceuticals (GSP) of CFDA by enterprises

Figure 6-3 The Distribution of GSP Deficiencies in Unannounced Inspections in Drug Circulation Field

	**Critical deficiencies	*Major deficiencies	Total	Proportion
General Provisions	35	0	35	16.99%
Quality Management System	0	8	8	3.88%
Institutions and Quality Management Responsibilities	0	17	17	8.25%
Personnel and Training	0	9	9	4.37%
Document of Quality Management System	5	6	11	5.34%
Facilities and Equipment	0	19	19	9.22%
Calibration and Verification	0	19	19	9.22%
Computer system	6	9	15	7.28%
Procurement	2	9	11	5.34%
Receipt and Acceptance Inspection	0	12	12	5.83%
Storage and Maintenance	0	23	23	11.17%
Sales	18	5	23	11.17%
Delivery	0	0	0	0.00%
Transport and Distribution	0	3	3	1.46%
After-sales Management	0	1	1	0.49%
Total	66	140	206	

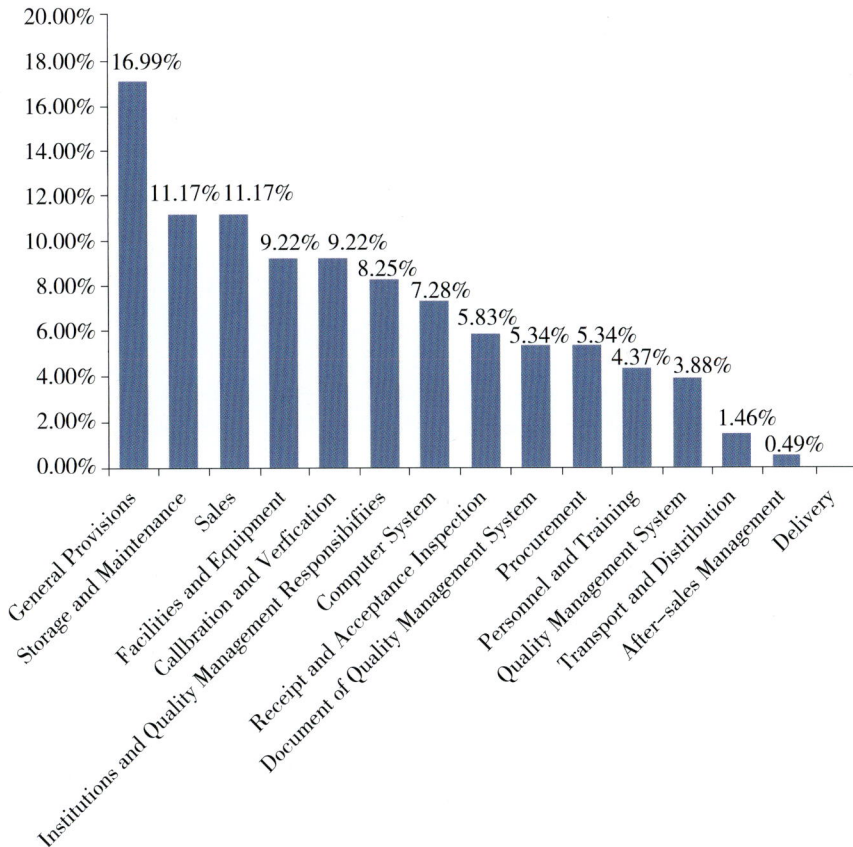

Figure 6-3 Distribution of the Deficiencies of GSP Violations by Enterprises

The GSP deficiencies of drug circulation enterprises mainly focused on the General Provisions, Storage and Maintenance, Sales. The main problems were:

(1) Fail to conduct business in accordance with the law and have false and cheating behaviors.

The enterprise changed the registered business address without authorization; established warehouses to store drugs beyond the scope of business license; provided conditions for illegal distribution of drugs; falsified the procurement source and sales flow of drugs; concealed bills and provided false materials; provided untruthful self-inspection report; falsified tax return; and tampered temperature and humidity monitoring data.

(2) Fail to store the drugs in accordance with regulations and fail to conduct effective monitoring and control of the temperature and humidity of warehouse.

(3) The bills, account, goods and payment was inconsistency for the purchase and sales of drugs, and the enterprise failed to implement national regulations for the sales of special medicines.

Chapter VII
GMP Observation Inspection by Foreign Organizations

I. Overview of Inspections

Based on the requirements in the letter from the Department of International Cooperation of China Food and Drug Administration, CFDI organized to complete 81 observation inspections on pharmaceutical manufacturers in 2016, involving 76 manufacturers, covering 20 provinces (municipalities) including Zhejiang and Shandong etc., of which Zhejiang, Shandong, Jiangsu, Guangdong, Hubei, Hainan and Hebei accounted for 80%, which was basically consistent with last year, but the proportion of each province showed a slight change.

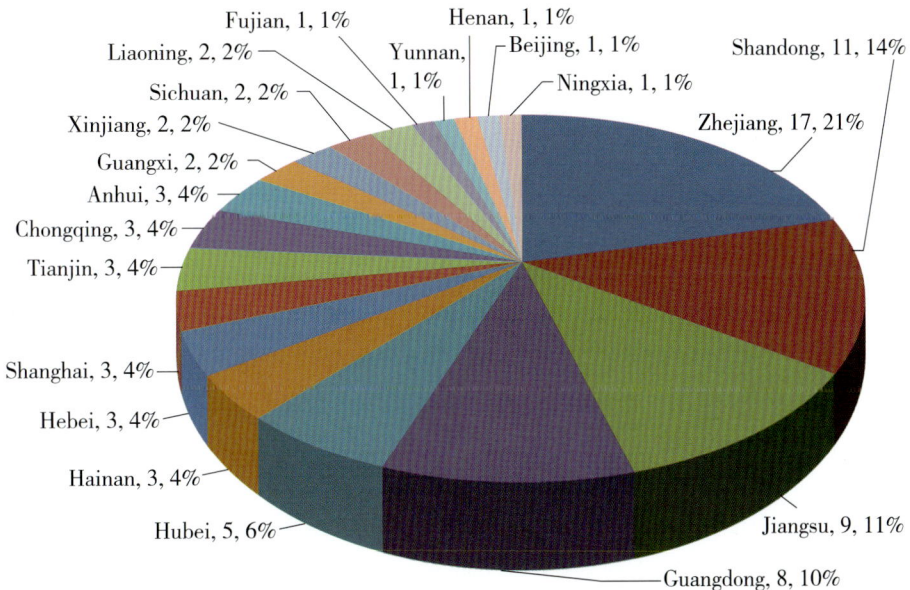

Figure 7-1　Distribution of Foreign Pharmaceutical Observation Inspections in Provinces (Municipalities) in 2016

In 2016, the inspection organizations involved in the observation inspection included 12 international organizations or foreign drug regulatory authorities, such as World Health Organization (WHO), European Directorate for Quality Medicines (EDQM), United States Food and Drug Administration (US FDA), Germany BGV, Agência Nacional de Vigilância Sanitária (ANVISA) and French National Agency for Medicines and Health Products Safety (ANSM). Nine pharmaceutical manufacturers were identified with critical deficiencies and failed the on-site inspections by foreign regulatory authorities / inspection organizations (accounting for 11%).

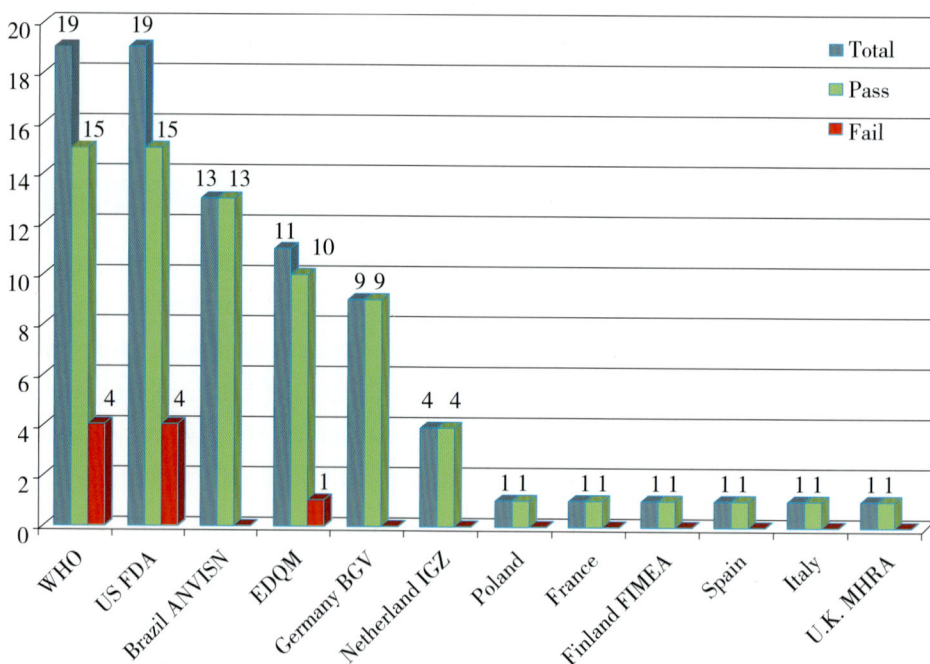

Figure 7-2　Fails in Foreign Pharmaceutical Observation Inspections in 2016

Compare with that in 2015, the fail rate was slightly increased. Among 9 enterprises failing in the inspection, most critical deficiencies involved the problems in data integrity (including conducting repeated tests until qualified, conducting tests after changing system time, deleting data, deleting the audit and tracking records, selectively using data, modifying the name of the electronic data, test sample injection, failing to record timely, untruthful records, loss of data and records, insufficient file record control, etc.), and some enterprises involved such aspects as unreasonably developed material standards and inadequate measures to avoid cross contamination. Overall, the problems in the data integrity is relatively prominent and were also the main reasons for the increase of fails of domestic enterprises in foreign inspections in 2016, which also reflects the change tendency of the current drug inspection.

The observation inspections this year involved a total of 172 drugs, including 119 APIs, 23 oral solid preparations, 19 injections, 5 biological products and 6 other products. Of the 81 inspections, there were 62 inspections involving APIs, accounting for 69%, and there were 12 inspections involving oral solid preparations, accounting for 13%. Of the drugs involved, APIs had the largest proportion, followed by oral solid preparations, and there was relatively less export of other dosage forms. Compared with that in 2015, the proportion of other dosage forms (including sterile products and biological products) receiving inspection increased, from 10% in 2015 to 18% in 2016.

Table 7-1   Distribution of Drug Types in the Inspections by Different Inspection Organizations

Inspection organizations		WHO	EDQM	US FDA	Germany BGV	Brazil ANVISA	Other organizations	Total
Drug types	APIs	27	12	53	14	10	3	119
	Oral solid preparations	14	0	2	1	2	4	23
	Injections	7	0	2	0	2	8	19
	Biological products	1	0	0	0	4	0	5
	Others	0	0	3	0	0	3	6
	Total	49	12	60	15	18	18	172

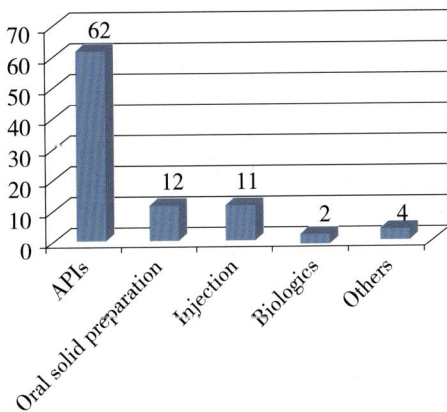

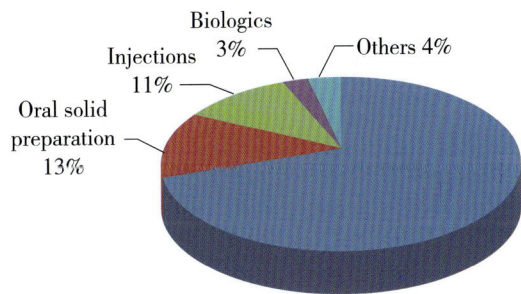

Distribution of the number of inspections in different dosage form   Distribution in different dosage form

Figure 7-3   Distribution of Inspections in Different Dosage Form

II. Main findings

The 1108 deficiencies were identified and recorded in the observation inspection in 2016. It was identified in the classification analysis on the deficiencies based on Chinese GMP (2010 version) that: the deficiencies in six categories including Quality Control and Quality Assurance, Documentation Management, Equipment, Materials and Products, Verification and Qualification and Premises and Facilities accounted for 88% of all the deficiencies. Compared with those in 2015, the deficiencies in Documentation Management increased from the 4th place to the second place in terms of its ranking and still showed an increase of 7% (from 10.5% to 17.3%) under an atmosphere that enterprises are gradually strengthening the management of data integrity, fully reflecting the concern extent and strict requirements for data integrity in currently foreign inspections.

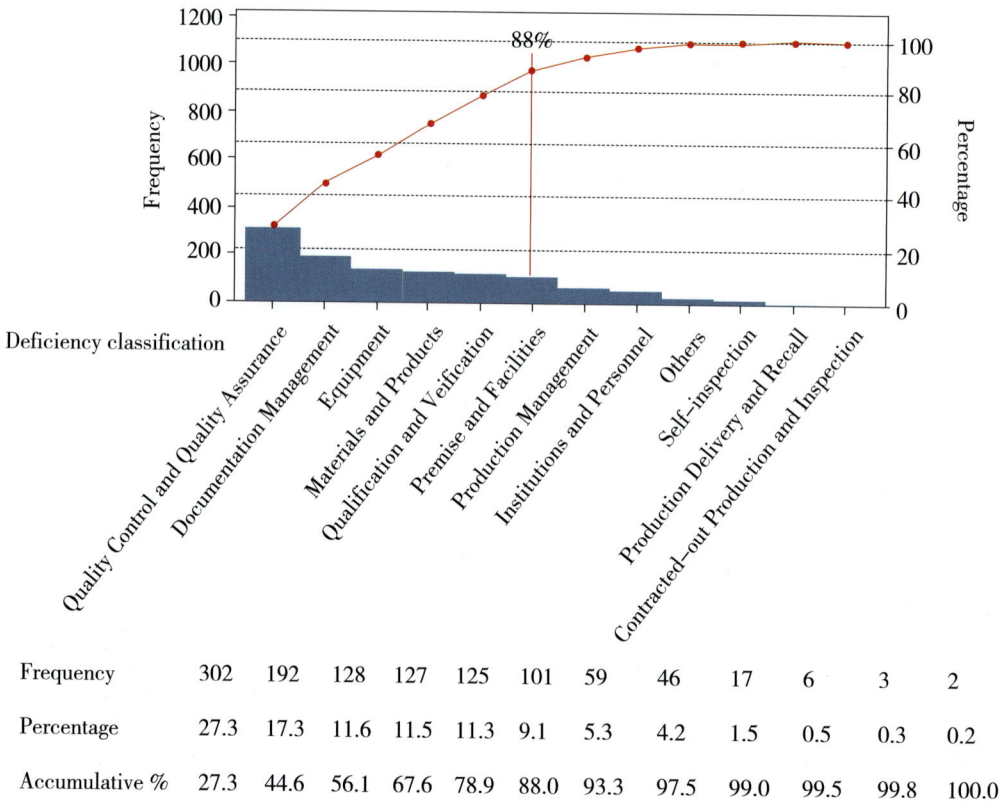

	Quality Control and Quality Assurance	Documentation Management	Equipment	Materials and Products	Qualification and Verification	Premise and Facilities	Production Management	Institutions and Personnel	Others	Self-inspection	Production Delivery and Recall	Contracted-out Production and Inspection
Frequency	302	192	128	127	125	101	59	46	17	6	3	2
Percentage	27.3	17.3	11.6	11.5	11.3	9.1	5.3	4.2	1.5	0.5	0.3	0.2
Accumulative %	27.3	44.6	56.1	67.6	78.9	88.0	93.3	97.5	99.0	99.5	99.8	100.0

Figure 7-4   Distribution of the Deficiencies Identified in Pharmaceutical GMP Observation Inspection by Foreign Organizations

In pharmaceutical GMP inspections by foreign organizations, the deficiencies in "Quality Control and Quality Assurance" topped the list, accounting for 27.3%. Main problems focused on the management of computerized analysis instruments in the laboratory, deviation handling and CAPA, product quality review, change control, OOS/OOT result processing, the laboratory's failing to meet the provisions for control procedure, microbial inspection management, quality risk management and stability test. The deficiencies in "Documentation Management" ranked the second, mainly focusing on four aspects including the completeness and traceability of records, life cycle management of documents, document completeness and record operation. The deficiencies in "Equipment" ranked the third, of which the deficiencies in the using and cleaning, calibration, maintenance and repair of equipment and water preparation system accounted for 83.6%. The deficiencies in "Materials and Products" focused on supplier management, identification of materials and products, process management of materials, compliance with material and product standards and release management. The deficiencies in "Verification and Qualification" mainly included the scientificity of validation, validation management and validation documents and records. The deficiencies in "Premises and Facilities" mainly included environmental control, management of storage area, the measures to prevent pollution and cross-pollution and life cycle management of premise and facilities.

III. Analysis on pharmaceutical GMP inspection of different organizations

In terms of inspection content, there was certain difference in the inspection focus among different pharmaceutical GMP inspection agencies, but it was found in the analysis on the deficiencies identified in the observation inspections in 2016 that there were relatively more deficiencies in six aspects including Quality Control and Quality Assurance, Documentation Management, Equipment, Materials and Products, Verification and Qualification and Premises and Facilities. As for the number of deficiencies in the final inspection report,

EDQM and WHO proposed more deficiency data, averaging 20 deficiencies in each inspection. For each deficiency, the problems identified during the inspection have been described. After the finish of inspection, such problems have been organized for preparing final inspection report (usually a month). US FDA proposed relatively less deficiencies in the inspections, averaging 7 deficiencies in each inspection, and did not take all the problems identified during the inspection as final deficiencies. The inspectors proposed the final deficiencies after the judgment based on the problems identified in combination with the product risks, and notify the enterprises in written form (Table 483) when holding the last inspection meeting.

(Note:The English version of this report is for reference only)